OTOLARYNGOLOGY RESEARCH ADVANCES

DYSPHAGIA

RISK FACTORS, DIAGNOSIS AND TREATMENT

OTOLARYNGOLOGY RESEARCH ADVANCES

Additional books in this series can be found on Nova's website
under the Series tab.

Additional E-books in this series can be found on Nova's website
under the E-book tab.

HUMAN ANATOMY AND PHYSIOLOGY

Additional books in this series can be found on Nova's website
under the Series tab.

Additional E-books in this series can be found on Nova's website
under the E-book tab.

OTOLARYNGOLOGY RESEARCH ADVANCES

DYSPHAGIA

RISK FACTORS, DIAGNOSIS AND TREATMENT

BRIAN S. SMITH
AND
MIKAEL ADAMS
EDITORS

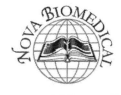

Nova Science Publishers, Inc.
New York

LIBRARY OF CONGRESS CATALOGING-IN-PUBLICATION DATA

Dysphagia : risk factors, diagnosis, and treatment / editors, Brian S. Smith and Mikael Adams.
    p. ; cm.
  Includes bibliographical references and index.
  ISBN 978-1-61942-104-2 (hardcover)
  I. Smith, Brian S. II. Adams, Mikael.
  [DNLM: 1. Deglutition Disorders. WI 250]

616.3'23--dc23

2011042521

Published by Nova Science Publishers, Inc. ✦ *New York*

Contents

Contents

Preface

Swallowing difficulties or dysphagia, can occur with numerous conditions, some of which are permanent, some reversible, and some progressive. The underlying etiology can be neurological, muscular, or mechanical/obstructive. The authors of this book present topical research in the study of the risk factors, diagnosis and treatment of dysphagia. Topics discussed include the etiology and prognosis associated with dysphagia; prevention of radiation-induced dysphagia; dysphagia in the myopathies; swallow screening as an essential component of acute stroke management and the perioperative risk factors for dysphagia.

Chapter I – The ability to swallow is essential for independent living, that is the ability not to take food supplements via non oral means. Swallowing difficulties (dysphagia) can occur with numerous conditions, some of which are permanent, some reversible and some progressive. The underlying aetiology can be neurological, muscular, or mechanical/ obstructive.

Chapter II – Swallowing dysfunction after radiotherapy for head and neck cancer is correlated with compromised quality of life, anxiety and depression, and can lead to life-threatening complications such as aspiration pneumonia. Because the risk of radiation-induced dysphagia is associated with the use of concomitant chemotherapy and accelerated fractionation schedules, its incidence has considerably increased in recent years. More and more, dysphagia is recognized as the dose-limiting toxicity of head and neck radiotherapy. Highly conformal radiation techniques, such as intensity-modulated radiotherapy, have been successfully applied to spare salivary glands from high-dose radiation and prevent permanent xerostomia. It is to be expected that limiting the dose to the critical swallowing structures will similarly reduce the incidence of dysphagia. However, several questions regarding which swallowing structures are essential, and what volume and dose constraints should be applied, remain to be answered.

Obviously, efficient swallowing is an extremely complex process, consisting of a series of coordinated events involving more than 30 pairs of muscles and 6 cranial nerves. Based on the physiology and anatomy of normal swallowing, a number of potential organs at risk for swallowing dysfunction have been identified. Correlating the dose to these structures with the presence of late dysphagia allows the definition of dose-response curves. However, it is not clear how the endpoint of dysphagia should be best described. Objective assessment is possible through invasive techniques such as videofluoroscopy with modified barium swallow or fiberoptic endoscopic evaluation of swallowing. There are also several validated questionnaires for subjective evaluation, such as the EORTC QLQ-HandN35 swallowing subscale, consisting of 4 questions regarding swallowing of liquid, swallowing of pureed food, swallowing of solid food, and aspiration when swallowing. Experience in the evaluation of xerostomia has indicated that patient-reported endpoints are preferable.

Despite the use of different dysphagia endpoints, different sets of potential organs at risk and different patient populations, results of published studies determining the critical structures for the prevention of swallowing complications are remarkably consistent. Apparently, both the mean dose to the pharyngeal constrictor muscles and the larynx, as well as the volume of those structures receiving 50 – 60 Gy, is significantly correlated with the occurrence of late dysphagia. These data imply that sparing these structures could prevent late dysphagia. However, no clear dose or volume constraints can yet be proposed, and currently, the best approach consists of keeping the radiation dose to these structures as low as possible. On the other hand, avoiding underdosing to the targets in the vicinity should remain the highest priority.

Chapter III – Myopathies are hereditary or acquired diseases of skeletal muscle that result from dysfunction of any constituent of this tissue, leading to the onset of isolated symptoms or combinations of signs and symptoms. There are several types of myopathies, among them inflammatory ones, muscular dystrophies, congenital myopathies, mitochondrial myopathies, and metabolic myopathies. Swallowing is a neurophysiological process whose main function is the efficient transport of food from the mouth to the stomach and which may be divided into four phases: preparatory, oral, pharyngeal, and esophageal. Dysphagia is defined as a set of alterations in any one of these phases, which may cause changes in eating pleasure, malnutrition, dehydration, and even the risk of death. Dysphagia is one of the changes that may be present in myopathies and may vary according to the type of myopathy and the duration of the disease, among other factors. It may appear as an initial symptom or during the course of the disease. Together with cerebrovascular accidents and cranial traumas, neuromuscular diseases are one of the main causes of dysphagia, mainly as a consequence of changes in skeletal muscle directly related to the swallowing process. Speech therapy intervention is essential for dysphagic patients in order to identify factors that increase the risk of tracheal aspiration and to determine ways of avoiding it, thus guaranteeing safe swallowing. This therapy starts with a process of clinical and instrumental evaluation of swallowing. Clinical evaluation is of fundamental importance and guides the indication of objective exams, when necessary, as well as the therapeutic process. Among the objective or complementary methods, videofluoroscopy of swallowing, nasofibrolaryngoscopy and manometry are those most frequently used. After clinical and complementary evaluation it is possible to make an appropriate speech therapy diagnosis and to establish a later conduct regarding the safest feeding route, as well as the indication of rehabilitation or management. Few studies of myopathies have described speech therapy rehabilitation in dysphagia, as well as its efficacy. As is the case for other neurological diseases, it should be kept in mind that the main objective of rehabilitation in the presence of dysphagia often is not the return to, or the maintenance of, feeding by the oral route, but rather the provision of safe nutrition and hydration conditions.

Chapter IV – Dysphagia following stroke is common and increases patient risk of poor outcomes and adverse events. Swallow screening is an important process of care for patients who suffer acute stroke. This brief examination aims to identify those patients that may be at risk of swallowing problems so that comprehensive assessment and management can be provided. However, despite wide agreement that swallow screening is an essential component of care, there is no agreement regarding how or when screening should be performed, and by whom. Debate continues regarding the validity and reliability of various screening tools, and whether they are able to provide an acceptable level of certainty in risk detection. The chapter reviews the current evidence underpinning swallow screening for acute stroke patients.

Published clinical quality audits on acute stroke populations have reported suboptimal compliance with swallow screening. Current evidence suggests that multiple factors contribute to screening compliance, including the structures and systems within health care facilities, such as stroke unit care. The provision of swallow screening may also be influenced by demographic and stroke-related variables of the patients themselves, such age, gender and stroke severity.

The results of the authors' recent research on the factors that influence the quality of stroke swallow screening will be presented. This was conducted in three Australian tertiary hospitals. The study retrospectively audited the care provided to 300 patients admitted with acute stroke. Data was collected on swallow screen compliance and other variables of interest including stroke unit admission, day of admission, patients' age, gender, English proficiency, comorbidities, pre-stroke levels of independence and type of accommodation, stroke severity and length of stay. Logistical univariate and multivariate stepwise regression analysis was undertaken to explore the determinants of screening compliance in this population. In the sample, patients with milder stroke, and those admitted over a weekend, were at increased risk of not receiving a swallow screen.

Swallow screening is an accepted care process in acute stroke management, despite ongoing debate regarding the best way to conduct the screening. Studies, including The authors' own, report suboptimal provision of swallow screening. The factors that influence swallow screening compliance may be complex and include variables within hospital systems, as well as variables related to the patient and their stroke.

Chapter V – Swallowing disorders are a significant cause of morbidity and mortality. Unrecognized dysphagia can lead to dehydration, malnutrition, aspiration pneumonia, or airway difficulty. The etiology is numerous and may be neurologic, muscular, or obstructive. Though many conditions may be associated with dysphagia, iatrogenic causes are also common. Anterior cervical spine surgery is often associated with varying degrees of post-operative swallowing difficulties. Understanding the risk factors as well as the anatomy and pathophysiology of swallowing should aid diagnosis, treatment, and limitation of dysphagia complications.

After identifying there is a swallowing problem, the anatomic region or involved phase should be recognized. History alone may be enough to detect an esophageal etiology, but oral and pharyngeal phase problems are best delineated by careful physical exam and diagnosis often aided by radiographic and laboratory studies. Once cause is identified, treatment is individualized based on structural and functional abnormalities. If underlying cause of dysphagia is not treatable, a combination of dietary modifications and swallowing therapy is often helpful. In some patients, enteral therapy may be necessary in the short term or long term in extreme cases in order to provide adequate nutrition.

Chapter VI – The clinical swallow examination (CSE) is often the only tool given to speech and language therapists to identify patients with a high risk of aspiration, penetration and dysphagia. With the help of the CSE, the clinician is able to gauge the oral phase. However, it is difficult to assess the pharyngeal phase because it is impossible see what is happening. Several studies report poor sensitivity – that is, the ability to identify true aspirators, and poor specificity – the ability to classify true nonaspirators. Even experienced clinicians can identify aspiration with the assessment of clinical parameters in only 40–60% of the radiologically verified examples. This is why the authors would be grateful for rapid and reliable methods and procedures that boost the sensitivity and specificity of the clinical assessment. Many publications propose several methods – one of them cervical auscultation (CA). In this article I am reviewing about 40 years of experience with and research on the knowledge of CA. The focus will be on studies employing the methodical basis of CA, acoustic analysis, or imaging techniques. Finally, I will discuss the diagnostic contribution of CA to the assessment of swallowing disorders and delineate further research prospects.

Chapter VII – Disorders of eating, drinking and swallowing (also known as 'dysphagia') commonly affect people with Down's syndrome (DS) across the lifespan. This is due to the influence of several factors, including the abnormal oral-facial features that are characteristic of the syndrome, as well as comorbid health conditions that impact on the safety and integrity of the swallowing process.

The relevant literature is consulted to explore aspects of the eating, drinking and swallowing process in people with Down's syndrome from birth onwards, and examine how this process differs from that in the general population.

Discussion focuses on how the typical eating, drinking and swallowing process in DS individuals is frequently associated with abnormal functioning of the swallowing mechanism at various levels, and how it can very often lead to dysphagia and its potentially life-threatening sequelae.

Finally, this paper considers the role of healthcare practitioners in the identification and management of dysphagia in individuals with DS, including implications for treatment planning and health service delivery.

In: Dysphagia
Editors: B. S. Smith and M. Adams

ISBN 978-1-61942-104-2
© 2012 Nova Science Publishers, Inc.

Chapter I

The Management of Dysphagia: A Clinical and Ethical View

*David G. Smithard**
Medical Director, Kent Community Health Trust, Trinity House,
Ashford, Kent, UK

The ability to swallow is essential for independent living, that is the ability not to take food supplements via non oral means. Swallowing difficulties (dysphagia) can occur with numerous conditions, some of which are permanent, some reversible and some progressive. The underlying aetiology can be neurological, muscular, or mechanical/ obstructive.

Dysphagia is not only determined by its aetiology but also by the site affected. Swallowing can be compromised by pathological processes within the oral cavity, pharynx, oesophagus and stomach. Other conditions can affect swallowing as a secondary effect eg severe lung disease, poor conscious level, and cognitive problems.

The aetiology and prognosis associated with dysphagia poses several problems. When to feed, who to feed and how to feed. What is the role of enteral feeding, does it help recovery in those reversible conditions eg stroke or does it just prolong life needlessly or is it appropriate in the general management of malignant conditions eg cancer, AIDS.

---

* Tel +44 (0) 1233 667842, Email david.smithard@kentcht.nhs.uk.

Decision making, therefore, has both a clinical and an ethical view point. Decisions need a multidisciplinary input, including where possible the patient, taking in to account previous expressed or documented views, prognosis and therefore the risk/benefit ratio of the intervention.

Swallowing is the act of transferring food/ liquid from the oral cavity to the stomach, where as eating is the act of transferring food from the plate to the mouth. Although appearing simple, swallowing is complex involving many muscles of the face, mouth, pharynx, larynx and oesophagus to occur safely. Not only this, cessation of respiration needs to occur in time with the pharyngeal swallow. This whole process has been called the most complex all or none reflex (1). The inability to hold a breath during a swallow, and exhale after a swallow, results in a compromised swallow with a risk of aspiration (2).

The ability to swallow food is neurologically complex, and much of the research has been undertaken using a single swallow model, where as frequently, particularly with fluids, there are multiple continuous swallows; for instance in a prolonged drink with multiple continuous swallows, the epiglottis (3) stands up an does not remain flat.

The neurological control of swallowing is as complex, if not more so, as the muscular control. The swallowing centre has bilateral representation within the pontine medullary junction. The hemispheric representation is widespread (amygdala, frontal, parietal lobes, insula, motor strip etc) (figure 1) and all though representation of the swallow is bilateral one hemisphere is frequently more dominant than the other (4-6).

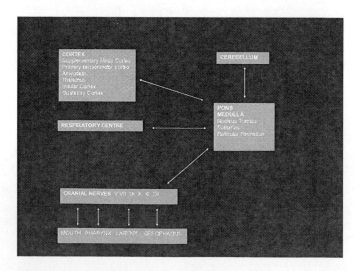

Figure 1. Neurological Control of swallowing.

Phases of Swallowing

Swallowing has three phases, oral, pharyngeal and oesophageal. Bolus preparation is the only part of the swallow that is voluntary, i.e. under control of the individual; the other phases once triggered occur reflexly. The various phases are sequential and coordinated with crucial timing. With increasing age this will still occur, however the leeway for error is reduced, and any slight change in timing could result in aspiration (7,8). Consequently any changes with the structure or control of any of these phases could result in dysphagia occurring. Dysphagia with or without overt aspiration exposes the individual to a risk of malnutrition infection and death (table 1). As a result, the primary aim of swallowing management, except that of removing the underlying aetiology, is to ensure safe nutrition.

Table 1. Complications of Aspiration

No effect
Coughing/ choking
Recurrent and often transient temperature
Wheeze
Oxygen Desaturation
Chest infection
Lung abscess
Chronic Obstructive Airways Disease
Malnutrition
Confusion
Fits secondary to hypoxia
Coma
Death

The swallow, is essentially, the passage of food and liquids through a series of muscular spaces/ tubes, which actively propel the bolus from the mouth to the oesophagus and thence the stomach. As a consequence anything that interferes with the function of this muscle will result in dysphagia and possible aspiration or even reflux. For the movement of the bolus to occur unhindered, there are essentially three conditions that need to be in place, firstly that the muscle works (ie the nerve supply is intact and the muscle tissue is functioning. A loss of nerve supply or muscle damage or both will result in dysphagia); secondly that there is no obstruction to the onward movement of the bolus; and thirdly there needs to be enough saliva to ensure that the mouth is not dry (8).

Oral Phase

The two of most important muscles associated with the oral phase of swallowing are the orbicularis oris (9) and the tongue The orbicularis oris is a composite muscle drawing fibres from surrounding facial muscles. The nerve supply is from branches of the facial nerve. Failure of the orbicularis oris to function with a dysfunction of the facial nerve as in stroke (upper motor neurone lesion) or Bell's palsy (lower motor neurone lesion) will result in a difficulty in closing the mouth and hence a difficulty with swallowing and or oral incontinence with dribbling and the loss of food out of the mouth.

Table 2. Medication affecting the ability to Swallow

Anticholinergic Medication - Dry Mouth
Amitryptaline
Toltoridine
Alpha Blockers
Calcium Antagonists
Dieuretics
Opiate Medication - Dry Mouth
Morphinie
Codiene
Medication affecting taste
Rifampicin
Metformin
Metronidiazole
Sedatives - Drowsiness
Benzodiazepines
SSRIs
Psychotropic Medication
Energy Intake and appetite reduced
Metformin,
Digoxin,
Corticosteroids,
TCAs

The tongue is a large muscle that is unusual in that it pushes rather than pulls. Nerve supply is via the XII cranial nerve. Loss of neural innervation will result in tongue weakness and hence difficulty in forming a bolus and then transmitting that bolus to the back of the mouth and into the pharynx. Motor neurone disease, stroke and malignancy are three conditions that affect tongue function.

Saliva is important in the ability to swallow. A dry mouth makes swallowing very difficult as any one who has attempted to eat cream crackers without a drink can testify. The amount of saliva present in all age groups is adequate unless there is a stress on the system. In older people this is frequently secondary to medication (see table 2) and in younger people, autoimmune disease such as Sjögren's Disease. Other causes include radiotherapy resulting is destruction of the salivary glands.

Infection with candida can affect all three phases of swallowing, causing pain. Treatment with nystatin of diflucan will usually resolve the problem. Fungal infections usually occur in immunocompromised patients (steroid use, chemotherapy, AIDs). Those using steroid inhalers for reversible airways disease may suffer with thrush if they fail to wash their mouth out after using the inhaler (8,10).

Pharyngeal Phase

Once food enters the pharynx the swallow will trigger. It had been dogma that the swallow would trigger once the bolus had passed the base of the faucial arches (11). Much of this evidence was gained from studying single isolated swallows, it is understood now that the swallow can trigger at some time after the base of the faucial arches. Prior to the commencement of the swallow the airway is protected by the vocal cords and elevation of the larynx; elevation of the soft palate and the anterior movement of the posterior pharyngeal wall protect the nasal passages and reflux through the nose (12).

Similarly to the oral phase, the pharyngeal phase can be affected by mechanical and neurological means. Mechanical issues may include a foreign body, extrinsic compression or intrinsic narrowing due to a stricture (benign or malignant), pharyngeal diverticulum. Neurological disease will include stroke, motor neurone disease, spasm of the upper oesophageal sphincter. Occasionally people will complain of a lump in the throat causing swallowing difficulties with no organic cause, this is globus hystericus. Some people present with total dysphagia, but on investigation no abnormalities are found, in this instance following investigation the ability to swallow usually recovers.

Oesophageal Phase

The oesophageal phase of swallowing is active and involves propulsion of the bolus down the oesophagus. The fact that it is active allows people to swallow safely whilst standing on their head.

Mechanical issues may include a foreign body, extrinsic compression or intrinsic narrowing due to a stricture (benign or malignant). Acid reflux due to an incompetent gastro-oesophageal sphincter has been noted to result in an abnormal pharyngeal transit and aspiration. Neurological disease is more unusual but includes mega oesophagus (abnormal myenteric plexi), presby oesophagus, and cork screw oesophagus.

Assessment

The clinical assessment of the ability to swallow safely, particularly in those with a neurological aetiology is that none of the bedside swallowing assessments are sensitive or specific enough (table 3) to reliably state aspiration is not occurring. There have been many studies over the years and work has been done to try and refine the bedside assessment with limited success (laryngeal auscultation, adding a chest radiograph to the bedside assessment, pulse oximetry) (13-16).

Table 3. Clinical Assessments of Swallowing

Bedside swallow assessments
3 oz Swallow Test
Timed Swallow Test
Bedside Swallowing Assessment / Screen
Additional Assessments not used routinely
Pulse Oximetry
Chest radiograph
Cervical auscultation

Following clinical assessment the standard radiological investigation is videofluoroscopy. Videofluoroscopy is the only investigation that provides information concerning the anatomy/ structure of the swallow, as well as the function of the swallow. However, patients are exposed to radiation, the equipment is not portable and patients may not be well enough to go to radiology. Despite videofluoroscopy being deemed the gold standard assessment, interpretation relies on the radiographer and agreement on the presence of aspiration may only be as high as 42% (17-19). Also, the assessment is being assessed at one time point, often with the person being assessed sitting in the ideal position being provided with controlled volumes to swallow. Feeding on the ward is often not optimal, may be rushed and sitting position incorrect.

Fibre optic nase endoscopy (20) does not expose people to radiation and can be done at the bedside. Operators need to be technically able, again single swallows are assessed and aspiration often has to be surmised. Operators have been known to duck as liquid passes the end of the endoscope. Increasingly the images a videoed and shown on a television screen and recorded to be reviewed at a later date. This has improved reporting. Other means of assessing the swallow are documented in table 4.

Table 4. Non Clinical Assessment of the ability to Swallow

Routine Assessments
Videofluoroscopy
Fibreoptic endoscopic evaluation of swallowing
Assessments used on occasions
Lateral cervical soft tissue radiography post contrast
Ultrasound
Pharyngeal or oesophageal manometry
Scintigraphy
Electromyography

Management

The primary aims of the management of dysphagia, after treating any reversible conditions, is to ensure that the person is being provided with enough calories. Lack of calories will ultimately result in death. The treatment choices will depend on the underlying aetiology and the prognosis relating to the aetiology. Many decisions may have a moral and or an ethical component, where frequently there is no right and wrong answer (21,22).

If there is a reversible condition (e.g. infection, poor mouth care) then the underlying cause needs to be treated or removed. Once this has happened then little else will need to be done. Normal feeding will resume and any supportive or supplemental feeding will be short term.

In many neurological cases the requirement for nutritional support will be medium to long term. Depending on the stage of the condition, whether the neurological deficit is fixed or potentially reversible the decision to be made is which type of enteral feeding should be used, and when (23).

Where the outcome will be death (AIDs, malignancy, dementia, motor neurone disease) the questions although similar are frequently more difficult, and the goals of feeding enterally may be different (24).

Methods of Providing Nutrition

There are two essential methods of providing nutrition: the first uses the gut and is termed enteral feeding, the second is via the vascular system and is termed parenteral.

Enteral Nutrition

Oral Feeding

Where possible any feeding should be via the oral route, using different consistencies of food and swallowing manoeuvres (table 5).

Sip feeds may increase total energy intake irrespective of whether the person is underweight (21). People with chronic disease may be able to use sip feeds and maintain their usual diet. The use of sip-feeds remains controversial because evidence for efficacy depends the disease group, in which their use has been studied. In stroke patients, their routine use, at this time cannot be supported (25), but where nutritional needs are such, and then they should be supplied. A similar argument exists for patients with dementia. The strongest evidence for the use of sip feeds, would appear for their use pre and post operatively for patients with a fractured neck of femur (26), but there is not universal agreement(27). Evidence is available for their use post operatively in abdominal surgery to reduce complication rates, but whether mortality or length of hospital stay are inflenced is open to debate (28). In the UK £350m is spent annually on sip feeds to treat malnutrition in the home setting (21). Unfortunately many people find the feeds unpalatable and wastage is frequently high (29). Reviews by Potter(30) have questioned their cost and clinical effectiveness

Table 5. Examples of strategies to aid oropharyngeal dysphagia

Disorder		Postural technique	Food consistency
Oral stage	Reduced tongue elevation	Tilt head back	Thin to thick fluids
	Reduced cheek tension	Tilt head to stronger side	Thin liquid to puree
Triggering of pharyngeal swallow	Delayed/ absent	Chin down	Avoid thin liquids
Pharyngeal stage	Unilateral pharyngeal weakness	Rotate head to weaker side	Liquids to thin puree
	Bilateral pharyngeal weakness	Lie down	Liquids to thin puree
	Reduced laryngeal elevation	Chin down	Thick liquid/ solids

Different food consistencies behave differently. The rheology varies which can result in dysphagia and aspiration occurring with specific foods. For instance thin liquids tend to disperse and are difficult to control and hold as discreet bolus; therefore if the tongue is not functioning liquids cannot be easily formed into a bolus, and may enter the pharynx before the airway is safe.

Often in the management of dysphagia (32), fluids are thickened. The basis of the premise is that the swallow is a problem, therefore aspiration is a risk, therefore pneumonia or even death may ensue. However, patients do not like there fluids thickened, drinks look like wall paper paste, evidence shows that fluid intake drops and there is a risk of dehydration and reduced survival (31). Rather than using proprietary thickeners it might be better to use fluid dense readily available foods such as thick soups (home made soup), yoghurt, thick custard etc.(33). Similarly, altering the consistency of food, e.g. liquidised or pureed, if not done well can make wholesome food look like cat food or worse, something the cat has already eaten.

One question that needs to be answered is that; are free fluids really hazardous, does aspiration of water matter, can the evidence available for stroke be extrapolated to other disease processes (34-36)? Are people aspirating or not when assessed at the bedside?

Enteral Nutrition

In those with more severe problems and those that cannot take food orally, enteral provision of nutrition needs to be considered. Enteral nutrition is frequently provided by nasogastric (NGT) or orogastric in the first instance, followed by gastrostomy (placed endoscopicaly, radiologically or surgically), the percutaneous endoscopic (PEG) route is the most common, tubes into the duodenum or beyond are occasionally used (37). An alternative, though less socially acceptable route, is rectal feeding (38). Long term use of enteral/Parenteral nutrition will result in disturbed appetite sensations (39), and can sometimes inhibit rehabilitation of the oral swallow as hunger is suppressed.

The greatest concerns centres around the increasing use of long term enteral feeding, is not only from a cost point of view, but also an ethical and moral point of view (discussed later). For instance the use of PEG placement has rocketed in the United States, from 15 000 in 1989 to 216 000 in 2006 (40,41), and in the UK £129m was spent in 2003 on prescribed artificial nutrition (21).

The method of enteral nutrition will depend on what is causing dysphagia. To provide calories in the short term, nasogastric tubes would be adequate providing they are managed appropriately. Longer term provision of nutrition is frequently provided via an enetrostomy. Enterostomy tubes may be placed with in the stomach or further down into the jejunum. The method of placement may vary; gastrostomy tubes are frequently placed via the percutanoeus route, where as jejunostmy tubes are placed radiologically. Both can be placed surgically. There are few problems associated with enterostomy feeding, though as they are an invasive procedure there is a small mortality risk (table 6+7) (42-44).

When using either a NGT or PEG, the aim is to provide nutrition, not to prevent aspiration. The risk of aspiration may actually increase, either by reduced pharyngeal transit, delayed triggering of the swallow, food sticking to the tube (if NGT is being used to supplement oral intake), increased oro-pharyngeal secretions and gastro-oesophageal reflux. With PEGs, Pump assisted feeding often results in less diarrhoea, less reflux, less aspiration and better glucose control compared to bolus feeding (44). NGT has an associated aspiration risk of 25-40% (40). Enteral tubes are not without their problems and both NGT and gastrostomy tubes carry significant morbidity and slightly less risk of mortality (table 7). These may be reduced by the use of specialist teams such as that described by Rimmer et al.(45).

Table 6. Complications of enteral feeding

Nasogastric Tube	Gastrostomy
Nasal alar ulceration Sinusitis Tracheobronchial fistuala Food sticking to tube Incompetent gastroesophageal sphincter Pulmonary oedema Mis placement of tube Aspiration pneumonia Gastric distress Diarrhoea Death	Skin excoriation Stomal leak Wound infection Fever Gastro oesophageal reflux Aspiration pneumonia Gastric distress Diarrhoea Peritonitis Gastro colic fistula Death

Table 7. Mortality after placement of enteral tubes

Study, y	Intervention	Type of Patient, No.	Outcome
Heimbach,[28] 1970	Surgical feeding tube	Neurogenic, 100	63% Mortality by 1 mo
Matino,[29] 1981	Jejunostomy tube	Neurogenic, 54	33% Mortality by 1 mo, 50% mortality among survivors by 6 mo
Golden et al,[30] 1997	PEG tube	Mixed population, 102	24% Mortality by 6 mo, 55% mortality by 2 y
Kaw and Sekas,[31] 1994	PEG tube	Mixed population, 46	20% Mortality by 1 mo, 59% mortality by 18 mo
Hull et al,[19] 1993	PEG tube	Mixed population, 49	8% Mortality by 1 mo, mean survival <6 mo
Kohli and Block,[20] 1995	PEG tube (review of 4 studies)	Mixed population, 612	16%-30% Mortality by 1 mo
Nevins,[21] 1989	PEG tube or gastrostomy tube	Neurogenic, 22	41% Mortality by 3 wks
Fay et al,[22] 1991	PEG vs nasoenteric tube	Mixed population, 109	50% Mortality by 4 mo for both populations
Hassett et al,[23] 1988	Gastrostomy tube	Neurogenic, 87	20% Mortality by 1 mo, 40% mortality by 1 y
Grant et al,[33] 1998	PEG tube or gastrostomy tube	Mixed population, 81 105	24% Mortality by 1 mo, 63% mortality by 1 y, 81.3% mortality by 3 y
Finocchiaro et al,[34] 1997	PEG tube	Mixed population, 136	9.5% Mortality by 1 mo, 58% mortality by 1 y, 65% mortality by 2 y
Loser et al,[35] 1998	PEG tube	Mixed population, 210	66% Mortality by 1 y
Fisman et al,[36] 1999	PEG tube	Mixed population, 175	18% Mortality by 30 d, 61% mortality by 1 y
Light et al,[36] 1995	PEG tube	Mixed population, 416	9% Mortality by 1 mo
Bergstrom et al,[35] 1995	Gastrostomy tube	Mixed population, 77	21% Mortality by 1 mo, 64% mortality by 1 y

*Neurogenic indicates dementia, cerebrovascular accident, trauma, anoxic brain injury, Parkinson disease, Guillain-Barré syndrome, or motor neuron disease; PEG, percutaneous endoscopic gastrostomy; and mixed population, patients with neurogenic mechanical disorders and cancer.

The two major complications of gastrostomy placement are infection, which can be reduced by the prophylactic use of broad spectrum antibiotics, and delayed gastric emptying and reflux, which can be managed with prokinetic drugs, but the long term efficacy of this has been questioned (28).

An alternative would be to place the tube into the jejunum.A PEG will need the appropriate management and support. In some, there will be an opportunity to remove it, and therefore a regular review is required (46,47). Carers need to be instructed on how to manage the tube, such as rotating it (depends on type) to prevent buried bumper syndrome, managing blockages and what to do if the tube falls out (37).

Enteral feeding also has its social consequences, the inability to enjoy food, not wanting to mix at meal times, which may result in isolation resulting in loneliness and possibly depression.

PEG vs NGT

Many patients find the NGT physically and psychologically uncomfortable. This may result in treatment failures. It is generally considered that a PEG is preferred over NGT for body image, however this not true for all, and in many cases the decision is a clinical one based on the time enteral feeding is likely to be required and treatment failure with the NGT. Placement of a PEG has serious psycho-social implications for both the patient and carer, and should not be performed without due care.

How long should a NGT be persevered with? The decisions made will depend on the person and their medical problem. In general a NGT should be persevered with for approximately four weeks, longer if tolerated, or if the underlying pathology resulting in dysphagia has resolving, or the use of the NGT is for supportive nutrition only.

The issue of PEG placement was usually raised by members of the medical team, with family members raising the issue in 1% of cases (41). The reason for the discussion and decision may be the need to discharge the patient and in some social situations a NGT cannot be managed, which may have more to do with the regulatory framework of Care Home registration and as a consequence the Care Home staff will not have the competence or confidence to manage, so a PEG is placed to facilitate discharge. The public often have the view that a PEG will result in a degree of clinical improvement, longevity and nutrition (48). The data, however shows that mortality at one year after PEG placement is 50% (49). Given these figures, the timing of any enterostomy is crucial, too soon and it may not be required (patient improves or dies) too late then there could be problems with malnutrition and refeeding syndrome, particularly if a compliance with other measures had been poor (50,51).

Parenteral Nutrition

Parenteral nutrition has little or no role to play in the management of dysphagia. Parenteral nutrition is required where there is failure of the gut, consequently in oro-pharyngeal dysphagia there is a functioning gut. If there is a delay whilst an enterostomy tube is to be placed then parenteral nutrition can be used to support the patient whilst awaiting the procedure. In these circumstances venous access is usually gained via peripheral line; longer term feeding would require central venous access.

Parenteral nutrition carries the added burden of frequent biological evaluation to ensure the correct nutrients are being provided, and there is a constant risk of septicaemia as there is a skin puncture with direct venous access.

Parenteral fluids are frequently used, appropriately in the acute phase of stroke or head injury (first 48 hours), any longer without extra calorific support will inhibit recovery, and may result in fluid overload.

Surgical Treatment

Over the years many different surgical techniques have been used in an attempt to prevent aspiration. This has included the epiglotopexy (52) and total laryngectomy (53).

Pharmacological Support

The first line pharmacological intervention in dysphagia is to stop those medications resulting in a dry mouth. Studies investigating the role of medication to rehabilitate the swallow are few. The use of nifedipine (54) controlled release in small study showed promise. Studies conducted in Japan have looked in to the role of ACE Inhibitors and have noticed a beneficial affect. It is proposed that the common pathway influenced by these medications, is via calcium channels, though substance P may play an important role (55).

Electrical/ Magnetic Stimulation

Over recent years work has been undertaken to investigate the role of Trans Cranial Magnetic Stimulation, oesophageal stimulation (56,57), palatal stimulation (58) and more recently pharyngeal stimulation. Palatal stimulation, involved the placing of electrodes on a plate to stimulate the elevation of the soft palate to close of the naso pharynx. There have only been small studies in this area and so far no clinical place has been identified.

Pharyngeal stimulation has hit the headlines with in the dysphagia field. The procedure known as Vita Stim has received a licence from the FDA, but many workers in the field doubt is efficacy. Studies by other workers have failed to support the findings of the original authors (59,60).

Trans Cranial Magnetic Stimulation is showing great promise. There is evidence that the effect of TCMS persists for up to one hour after a stimulation and that the swallow is improved. There is still a long way to go before this will reach the bedside.

Ethical Dilemmas

Dilemmas arise in the management of people/ patients when a belief system comes up against a treatment request that causes a conflict between the two. These situations arise, to a greater or less degree, in all areas of medicine. The ability to make a decision will lie in the ability and confidence of the attending clinicians to accept uncertainty and risk.

The over riding principle in health care is to have respect for the patient, this forms the cornerstone of an ethical approach and consists of two strands;

1) Autonomy; the ability to make choices, to make life your own, to have independent control of your identity.
2) Welfare; a concern for well being as apposed to an over bearing suffocating paternalistic/ maternalistic approach.

Although life can be physiologically sustained with artificial nutrition and hydration, there is no evidence that quality of life is improved (on balance it is usually made worse by artificial feeding) and no improvement in primary pathology can be expected. An ethical dilemma arises when there is a perceived conflict in duty to the patient. All human life has a worth, however the sanctity of life, although is important, should not be the be all and end all [see the Lancet 2005;366].

There is an ethical obligation to provide artificial nutrition and hydration based upon medical need, medical appropriateness and potential benefit (49,61). However, the duty of care to one will need to be balanced against the care of the many. Harris has argued that if a life is not possible to be lived independently, is it a life at all (62)? Therefore if there is no accepted life, there is no need to intervene. This all comes down to what is life, who can decide who keeps theirs?

At present, in the United Kingdom, there is much debate about the provision of nutrition to patients with brain injury. The arguments regarding feeding can be transferred to other causes of dysphagia so long as the different disease processes and prognoses are taken in to account. A balance needs to be struck between the prevention of death and the postponement of the inevitable. In many situations the decisions are straightforward and are not contentious, in some other situations, however, the person is neither dying nor rapidly medically improving. It is these patients that present moral and ethical dilemmas. What should be done? Can nutrition be used as part of palliative care? In this situation is death postponed, or is it more comfortable? If a competent person requests a medical treatment or in this situation desires to be fed, that could result in death being postponed, it is generally considered appropriate to refuse treatment if the consensus of medical opinion is that providing that treatment is futile. If death is imminent within days or a few weeks this may be appropriate, but what if death is a month or two months hence, does refusal to provide nutrition constitute murder (63,64).

Food does not only have a physiological and metabolic role, ie it provides fuel and essential nutrients for the body, but it fulfils a wider societal role. Food is used as a sign of friendship and hospitality. The failure to provide food or nutrition is very emotive and this leads into the discussion about whether the provision of food and enteral nutrition are the same. One point, however, is clear cut: doing nothing is not an option and will result in the death of the individual, but the provision of nutrition may not be of benefit. It is in this situation that the cost benefit (burden) ratio for the patient needs to be considered. Lennard-Jones(65) suggested that enteral nutrition, and accepted this, in many countries is the legal situation (49,66-68), is a treatment much the same as antibiotics and can be started and used as a trial of treatment, stopping when there has been no improvement (67). This is the position of the UK medical and nursing organizations (67). However, how can the success of enteral nutrition be assessed over a short period of time? What would be assessed/ measured? How can quality of life be assessed? Angus has suggested using life expectancy (>4 weeks) (49), life quality (whose (69)), weight gain and biochemical markers. Could we be better at selecting those for a PEG?

The provision of enteral nutrition requires consent, but often this is assumed to have been given for the passing of a NGT (implied consent), unless it is refused or resisted. What might a refusal mean in an ill and or confused patient? What statement is being made by the patient who persistently removes the NGT, this may be as high as 42% (70) of tubes placed. NGT removal may lead to recurrent replacement and, depending on local policies repeated exposure to radiological radiation. How should this be interpreted? Is removal deliberate or accidental?

Nasogastric tubes are resisted or repeatedly removed for a myriad of reasons, is it a statement of intent. In the case of brain injury the tube may be on the neglect side and is found by chance and is pulled due to a lack of understanding particularly if there is concurrent cognitive impairment (acute or long standing). Discomfort is another reason why tubes are removed (68). People with cognitive impairment may not understand why some one is approaching them with a tube and may be frightened of the impending "attack" and therefore push the perpetrator away (66,68).

If the wider team feel it appropriate, how should it be retained. Various methods have been put forward include a spacing device between thumb and index finger, nasal loop or bridle (70-74) or American football helmet (75). Does the use of restraint constitute a deprivation of liberty?

The insertion of a PEG requires careful consideration and formal informed consent. How can we be sure that informed consent has been obtained, especially in the cognitively impaired or dysphasic patient? What is the purpose of inserting the PEG, what are the goals that are hoping to be achieved? What is quality of life and whose quality of life is being considered? What is the best interests of the patient? What about autonomy (the right to control one's personal destiny (76)? What about capacity? All patients will need to be considered competent, ie have capacity unless proven otherwise, and this will need to be reassessed when ever a major decision needs to be made as capacity is decision dependent (77). Assessing some ones capacity is not just about a clinician deciding in isolation what is in a patients best interest, it is a about a conscious effort to understand what the patient's wishes are. Is it perverse that the patient ahs the right to refuse treatment but not the right to demand it? A lack of ability to communicate at all is deemed not to be competent. Capacity must be assumed until proven otherwise (78).

Increasingly in many countries the advanced directive/ living will, first considered in the 1960s (79,80) is becoming common place, it is suggested that specific inclusion of the use of artificial nutrition and hydration should be encouraged (80). Alternatives include the nomination of a proxy, and in England and Wales this person would be called a Lasting Power of Attorney (Welfare). In the situations where there is conflict an independent arbiter or advocate can be appointed to gather all information and produce a report written to express the best interests of the patient. One major decision that drives this process is the time frame that the treatment or intervention needs to happen. Frequently, in the case of the provision of enteral nutrition, an immediate decision is not required but neither can there be a delay of many weeks. It is imperative that the appropriate decision is made right at the beginning to avoid legal complications at a later date. However, the acceptance of advanced directives and how the influence decision making may vary with the clinician (81,82).

What about those patients/ people who are assessed as being at risk of aspiration because of a delayed or absent swallow, yet refuse enteral support in favour of continuing to eat their regular diet. The same discussions need to be had about their competency to make that decision, bearing in mind if they are able to understand and have the capacity to refuse enteral feeding then; surely, they have the capacity to decide to eat (table 8).

Table 8. Assessment of Capacity

Encourages participation of the patient
Identifies the relevant circumstances
Finds out the persons wishes, feelings, beliefs, and values
Avoids discrimination
Assess whether capacity will be regained and when
Protects the patient that any decision regarding life sustaining treatment is not motivated to hasten death or prejudges quality of life
Consults others
Avoids restriction of rights
Takes all the above into account when coming to a decision

Regnard and Louw 2011.

The cornerstone for any intervention is consent and hence the capacity to provide consent. Often capacity is difficult to define, but it mirrors that or the ability to consent, "the ability to understand information, manipulate it, come to a decision and to provide a reasoned argument for that decision". Lack of communication, refusal to agree to the medical plan or to cooperate with an assessment of capacity does not demonstrate a lack of capacity (79,83).

When some one lacks capacity, particularly in the short term, due to lack of consciousness, infection, drowsiness, or acute confusion / delirium, then advice needs to be sought form others to guide the decision making process. Despite the law providing people with a legal right to make decisions regarding treatment, no one can legally provide consent for a third party. Any decision must be made in a person's best interest taking into account previously expressed wishes/ statements, knowledge of the person, and likely outcome of the intervention (62).

Refusal to eat may be the only remaining control that some one has after a major brain injury or illness, or because of oral infection or dehydration, depression or the simple fact that the patient is dying. If treatment is refused, but then forcibly provided, this may be deemed "battery"(84), often it is considered appropriate to allow some one to die if they decide not to eat, but it is unethical to inform them that this is an option.

The medical profession and other care providers may need to be persuaded that persistent failure to eat is a terminal event in irreversible progressive brain failure, and is equivalent to other organ system failures that result in death (85,86).

It is important that the patient's "family" are informed that the withdrawal of nutrition and hydration does not mean the withdrawal of care, but the beginning of end of life care (Liverpool care pathway) (87). It may well be that the family need to be given "formal" permission to make the decision to choose palliation, but at the same time do not force decision making on to those that do not want it. Patients should continue to be treated with dignity. Pain should be controlled and suffering relieved. It should also be made known, that during the terminal phase of life, the death without intravenous fluids can peaceful and pain free. What we conceive as life may have been considered intolerable and undignified suffering by the patient. In the United States, where pro-life forces are extremely active, laws now exist to ensure that previously stated patient preferences regarding all medical and life-sustaining treatments are honoured.

Finally, we must consider whom we are treating: the patient, the family or our selves? Whatever decisions are made must be for the benefit/ good of the patient; often, however, they are made for the good of families or staff, and this is not acceptable. Whatever decision is made, it must be done after consultation with the relatives and the multidisciplinary team and after this be communicated with all staff, and that a decision not to feed will result in death.

At the end of the day the bottom line is that every human being of adult years and who has been determined to have the capacity to make an informed decision has the moral and legal right to determine what shall be done with their own body.

References

[1]   Doty,R.W. *Influence of stimulus pattern on reflex deglutition.* American Journal of Physiology 1951;166: 142-158.

[2]   Selley,W.G., Flack,F.C., Ellis,R.E. and Brooks,W.A. *Respiratory patterns associated with swallowing: Part 2; Neurologically impaired dysphagic patients.* Age and Ageing 1989;18: 173-176.

[3]   Dodds WJ, Stewart ET, Logemann JA. *Physiology and radiology of oral and pharyngeal phases of the normal swallow.* Am J Roent 1990;154:953-963.

[4]   Smithard DG. *Swallowing and stroke: neurological function and recovery.* Cerebrovascular Diseases 2002;1-8.

[5]   Hamdy,S., Aziz,Q., Rothwell,J.C., Singh,K.D., Barlow,J., Hughes,D.G., Tallis,R.C. and Thompson,D.G. *Nature Medicine* 1996;2:1217-1224.

[6]   Mosier,K., Patel,R., Liu,W-C., Kalnin,A., Maldjian,J. and Baredes,S. *Cortical representation of swallowing in normal adults: Functional implications.* Laryngoscope 1999;109:1417-1423.

[7]   Robbins,J., Hamilton,J.W., Lof,G.L. and Kempster,G.B. *Oropharyngeal swallowing in normal adults of different ages.* Gastroenterology 1992;103: 823-829.

[8]   Kendall KA, Leonard RJ,McKenzie S. *Common medical conditions in the elderly inpatient on pharyngeal bolus transit.* Dysphagia 2004;19:71-77.

[9]   Williams PL, Warwick R. editors *Gray's Anatomy 36th Edition.* Churchill Livingstone. London. 1980.

[10]   Smithard DG*Elderly patients and asthma.* Asthma Care Today 1994: 3(1): 8-9.

[11]   Perlman AL, Schultz JG, and VanDaele DJ. *Effects of age, gender, bolus volume and bolus viscosity on oropharyngeal pressure during swallowing.* J Appl Physiol 75: 33–37, 1993.

[12] Smithard DG*Dysphagia following stroke.* Reviews in Clinical Gerontology 1999; 9:81-93.

[13] Ramsey DJC and Smithard DG. *Assessment and Management of Dysphagia.* Hospital Medicine 2004

[14] Ramsey DJC, Smithard DG, Kalra L. *Silent Aspiration: what do we know?* Dysphagia 2006;20:218-225

[15] Collins,M.J. and Bakheit,A.M. *Does pulse oximetry reliably detect aspiration in dysphagic stroke patients.* Stroke 1997; 28(9):1773-1775

[16] Cardoso MCdeAF, Fontoura EG. *Value of the cervical auscultation in patients affected by neurogenic dysphagia.* Int Arch Otolaryngol 2009:13;431-439

[17] Scott,A, Perry,A. and Bench,J. *A study of interrater reliability when using videofluoroscopy as an assessment of swallowing.* Dysphagia 1998;13:223-227

[18] Ekberg,O., Nylander,G., Frans-Thomas,F., sjoberg,S., Birch-Jensen,M. and Hillarys,B. *Interobserver variability in cineradiographic assessment of pharyngeal function during swallow.* Dysphagia 1988;3:46-48.

[19] Smithard,D.G., O'Neill,P.A., Park,C., Morris,J., Wyatt,R., England,R. and Martin,D.F. *Complications and outcome after acute stroke: Does dysphagia matter.* Stroke 1997;27:1200-1204.

[20] Leder SB, Acton LM, Lisitano HL, Murray JT. *Fibreoptic endoscopic evaluation of swallowing (FEES) with and without blue dyed food.* Dysphagia 2005; 20:157-162.

[21] Stratton RJ. *Elucidating effective ways to identify and treat malnutrition.* Proc Nutr Soc 2005;64:305-1311

[22] Potter JM, Roberts MA, McColl JH, Reilly JJ. *Protein energy supplements in unwell elderly patients – a randomized controlled trial.* JPEN 2001;25:323-329.

[23] Blandford G, Watkins LB, Mulvihill MN, Taylor B. *Assessing abnormal feeding behavior in dementia: a taxonomy and initial findings.* In Research and Practice in Alzheimer's Disease. *"Weight loss and eating behavior in Alzheimer's Disease".* Eds Vellas B, Riviere A, Fitten J. 1998 Serdi, Paris and Springer Publishing. Pp 49-65

[24] Crotty B, McDonald J, Mijch AM, Smallwood RA. *Percutanoeous endoscopic gastrostomy feeding and AIDS.* J GAstroenterol Hapatol 2008;13:371-375

[25] *The   FOOD   Trial   Collaboration.   Routine   oral   nutritional supplementation for stroke patients in hospital (FOOD): a Multicentre randomized controlled trial.* Lancet 2005;365:753-763.

[26] Blundell JE, Stubbs RJ. *High and low carbohydrate and fat intakes: limits imposed by appetite and palatability and their implications for energy balance.* Eur J Clini Nutr 1999;53(S1):S148-S165.

[27] Espaulella J, Guyer H, Diaz-Escriu F, Mellado-Navas JA, CAstells M, Pladevall M. *Nutritional supplementation of elderly hip fracture patients: A randomized double-blind placebo-controlled trial.* Age and ageing 2000;295:425-431.

[28] National Institute for Clinical Excellence. *Nutrition Support for Adults.* National Collaborating Centre for Acute Care, Royal College of Surgeons, London. August 2006.

[29] Gosney M. *Are we wasting money on food supplements in elder care wards?* J Adv Nursing 2003;43:275-280.

[30] Potter JN, Langhorne P, Roberts M. *Routine protein energy supplementation in adults: systematic review.* BMJ 1998;317:495-501.

[31] O'Neill,P.A., Faragher,E.B., Davies,I., Mears,R., McLean,K.A. and Fairweather, D.S. *Reduced survival with increasing plasma osmolality in elderly continuing-care patients.* Age and Ageing 1990;19: 68-71.

[32] Odderson JR, Keaton KC, M^CKenna BS. *Swallow management in patients on an acute stroke pathway: Quality is cost effective.* Arch. Phys. Med. Rehabil. 1995;76:1130-1133.

[33] Vivanti AP, Campbell KL, Michelle S, Hannan-Jones MT, Hulcombe JA. *Contribution of thickened drinks, food, and enteral and parenteral fluids in hospitalised patients with dysphagia.* J Huim Nutr Diet 2009;22:148-155.

[34] Hinchey JA, Shephard T, Furie K, Smith D, Wang D, Tonn S. *Formal dysphagia   screening   protocols   prevent   pneumonia.*   Stroke 2005;36:1972-1976.

[35] Karagiannis MJP, Chivers L, Karagiannis TC. *Effects of oral intake of water in patients with oropharyngeal dysphagia.* BMC Geriatrics 2011;11(9).

[36] Garon BR, Engle M, Ormiston C: *A randomized control study to determinethe effects of unlimited oral intake of water in patients with identifiedaspiration.* J Neuro Rehab 1997, 11:139-148.

[37] Klor,B.M. and Milianti,F.J. *Rehabilitation of neurogenic dysphagia with percutaneous endoscopic gastrostomy.* Dysphagia 1999;14:162-164.

[38]   Bastin HC. A treatise on aphasia and other speech defects. HK Lewis, London 1898.

[39]   Elia M. *Hunger Disease* Clin Nutr 2000;19:379-386.

[40]   Baskin WN *Acute complications associated with bedside placement of feeding tubes.* Nutrition in Clinical Practice 2006;21:40-55.

[41]   Callahan CM, Haag KM, Buchanan NN, Nisi R. *Decision-making for percutaneous endoscopic gastrostomy among older adults in a community setting.* JAGS 1999;47:1105-1109.

[42]   Pearce CB, Duncan HD. *Enteral feeding Nasogastric, nasojejunal, percutaneous endoscopic gastrostomy, or jejunostomy: its indications and limitations.* Postgrad Med J. 2002;78:198-2004.

[43]   McMahon MM, Hurley D, Kamath PS, Mueller PS. *Medical and ethical aspects of long term enteral tube feeding.* Mayo Clin Proc. 2005;80:1461-1476.

[44]   Shang E, Geiger N, Sturm JW, Post S. *Pump-assiisted enteral nutrition can prevent aspiration in bedridden percutaneous endoscopic gastrostomy patients.* JPEN 2004;28:180-183.

[45]   Rimmer E, Berner YN, Gindin J, Barr DD, Levy S. *Low complication rate after percutaneous endoscopic gastrostomy by a geriatrics orientated team.* JAGS 1999;47:765-766.

[46]   Chong VH, Vu C. *Percutaneous endoscopic gastrostomy outcomes: can patient profiles predict mortality and weaning?* Singapore Med J. 2006;47:383-387.

[47]   Crarey MA, Groher ME. *Reinstituting oral feeding in tube fed adult patients with dysphagia.* Nutrition in Clinical Practice 2006;6:576-586.

[48]   Mitchel SC, Kiely DK, Lipsitz LA. *Does artificial enteral nutrition prolong the survival of institutionalised elders with chewing and swallowing problems?* J Gerontol Med Sci 1998;53A:M207-M213.

[49]   Angus F, Burakoff R. *The percutaneous endoscopic gastrostomy tubes: medical and ethical issues in placement.* Am J Gastroenterol 2003;98:272-277.

[50]   The FOOD Trial Collaboration. *Effect of timing and method of enteral tube feeding for dysphagic stroke patients (FOOD): a Multicentre randomized controlled trial.* Lancet 2005;365:764-772.

[51]   Kurien M, Sanders DS. *Improving outcomes following percutaneous endoscopic gastrostomy (PEG)- a seven day waiting policy is essential.* Clin Med 2011;11:411.

[52]   Brookes GB, McKelvie P. *Epiglottopexy: a new surgical technique to prevent intractable aspiration.* Ann Roy Coll Surg Engl 1983;293-296.

[53] Cannon CR, McLean WC. *Larngectomy for chronic aspiration.* Am J Otolaryngol 1982;3:1145-149.

[54] Perez,I., Smithard,D.G., Davies,H. and Kalra,L. *Pharmacological treatment of dysphagia in stroke.* Dysphagia 1998;13:12-16.

[55] Smithard DG *Substance P and swallowing after stroke.* Therapy 2006;3:291-298

[56] Hamdy S, Rothwell M, Aziz Q, Thompson DG. *Organization and reorganization of the human motor cortex: implications for recovery after stroke.* Clin Sci 2000;99:151-157

[57] Hamdy S, Rothwell JC, Aziz Q, Singh KD, Thompson D. *Long term reorganization of human motor cortex driven by short term sensory stimulation.* Nature Nueroscience 1998;1:64-68.

[58] Park CL, O'Neill PA, Martin DF. *A pilot exploratory study of oral electrical stimulation on swallow function following stroke: An innovative technique.* Dysphagia 1997;12:161-166.

[59] Logemann JA. *The effects of VitalStim a clinicl and research utility in dysphagia.* Dysphagia 2007;22·11-12.

[60] Ludlow CL, Humbert I, Saxa K, Poletto C, Sonies B, Crajido L. *Effects of surface electrical stimulation both at rest and during swallowing in chronic pharyngeal dysphagia.* Dysphagia 2007;22:1-10

[61] Regnard C, Leslie P, Crawford H, Matthews D, Gibson L. *Gastrostomies in dementia: bad practice or bad evidence?* Age and Ageing 2010;39:282-284.

[62] Harris J. *Consent and end of life decisions* J Med Ethics 2003;29:1-10.

[63] 101. The A-M, Pasman R, Onwuteaka-Philipsen B, Ribbe M, van der Wal G. *Withholding the artificial administration of fluids and food from elderly patients with dementia: ethnographic study.* BMJ 2002;325:1326-1330.

[64] Pasman HRW, Onwuteaka-Philipsen BD, Kriegsman DMW, Ooms ME, Ribbe MW, van der Wal G. *discomfort in nursing home patients in whom artificial nutrition and hydration is forgone.* Arch Intern Med 2005;165:1729-1735.

[65] Lennard-Jones. *Giving or withholding fluid and nutrients.*: ethical and legal aspects. J Roy Coll Physicians 1999;3:39-45.

[66] General Medical Council. *Withholding and withdrawing life-prolonging treatments: Good practice in decision-making.* GMC London 2002.

[67] British Medical Association. *Withholding and withdrawing life-prolonging treatment.* BMJ Books. London, 1998.

[68] Gillick MR. *Rethinking the role of tube feeding in persons with advanced dementia.* NEJM 2000;342:206-210.

[69] Carey JS. *Motor Neuron Disease: a challenge to medical ethics.* J Roy Soc Med 1986;79:216-220.

[70] Carrion MI, Ayuso D, Marcos M, Robles MP, de la Cal M, Alia I, Estean A. *Accidental removal of endotracheal and nasogastric tubes and intravascular catheters.* Critical Care Medicine 2000;28:63-66.

[71] Della Faille D, Hartoko T, Vandenbroucke M, Brands C, Schmelzer B, de Deyn PP. *Fixation of nasogastric tubes in agitated and uncooperative patients.* Rev Laryngol Otol Rhinol (Bord) 1998;119:59-61.

[72] Anderson MR, O'Connor M, Mayer P, O'Mahoney D, Woodward J, Kane K. *The nasal loop provides an alternative to percutaneous endoscopic gastrostomy in high-risk dysphagic stroke patients.* Clin Nutr 2004;23:501-506.

[73] Popovich MJ, Lockrem JD, Zivot J. *Nasal bridle revisited: an improvement in the technique to prevent unintentional removal of small-bore nasoenteric feeding tubes.* Critical Care Medicine 1996;24:429-431.

[74] Bevan J, Conroy SP, Harwood R, Gladman JRF. et al. *Does looped nasogastric tube feeding improve nutritional delivery for patients with dysphagia after acute stroke? A randomised controlled trial.* Age and Ageing 2010;39:624-30.

[75] Levine JA., Morris JC. *The use of a Football Helmet to secure a nasogastric tube.* Nutrition 1995;11:285.

[76] Oyebode F. *The Mental Capacity Act 2005.* Clin Med 2006;6:130-131.

[77] Hotopf M. *The assessment of mental capacity.* Clin Med 2005;5:580-584.

[78] Shickle D. *Mental Capacity Act 2005.* Clin Med 2006;6:169-173.

[79] Regnard C, Louw S. *Embedding the Mental Capacity Act into clinical practice in England and Wales.* Age and Ageing 2011;40:416-418.

[80] Gillick MR. *The use of advanced care planning to guide decisions about artificial nutrition and hydration.* Nutrition in Clinical Practice 2006;21:126-133.

[81] Bond CJ, Lowton K. *Geriatricians' views of advanced decisions and their use in clinical care in England: a qualitative study.* Age and Ageing 2011;40:450-456.

[82] Davidson KW, Hackler C, Caradine DR, McCord RS. *Physicians' attitudes on advance directive.* JAMA 1989;262:2415-2419.

[83] Finucane TE, Christmas C, Travis K. *Tube feeding in patients with advanced dementia. A review of the evidence.* JAMA 1999;282:1365-1370.

[84] Johnston C, Slowther A. *Ethical Issues: End of Life Issues.* www.ethox.or.uk/Ethics/eendoflife.htm.

[85] Flather-Morgan A. *Caring for patients with dysphagia: some ethical considerations.* SIG 13 Swallowing and Swallowing Disorders 1994;3:8-11.

[86] Lerner BH, Milkes D. *Teaching ethics to medical students.*

[87] Ellershaw J, Smith C, Overill S, Walker S, Aldridge J. Setting standards for symptom control in the last 48 hours of life. *J Pain and Symptom Management* 2001;21:2-17.

In: Dysphagia
Editors: B. S. Smith and M. Adams

ISBN 978-1-61942-104-2
© 2012 Nova Science Publishers, Inc.

Chapter II

Prevention of Radiation-Induced Dysphagia

Piet Dirix * *and Sandra Nuyts*

Department of Radiation Oncology, Leuvens Kankerinstituut (LKI),
University Hospitals Leuven, campus Gasthuisberg,
Leuven, Belgium

Abstract

Swallowing dysfunction after radiotherapy for head and neck cancer is correlated with compromised quality of life, anxiety and depression, and can lead to life-threatening complications such as aspiration pneumonia. Because the risk of radiation-induced dysphagia is associated with the use of concomitant chemotherapy and accelerated fractionation schedules, its incidence has considerably increased in recent years. More and more, dysphagia is recognized as the dose-limiting toxicity of head and neck radiotherapy. Highly conformal radiation techniques, such as intensity-modulated radiotherapy, have been successfully applied to spare salivary glands from high-dose radiation and prevent permanent xerostomia. It is to be expected that limiting the dose to the critical swallowing structures will similarly reduce the incidence of dysphagia.

* Corresponding author: Piet Dirix Department of Radiation Oncology, Tel + 32 16 34 76 00, Leuvens Kankerinstituut (LKI); Fax + 32 16 34 76 23, University Hospitals Leuven, campus Gasthuisberg, e-mail: piet.dirix@uzleuven.be, Herestraat 49, 3000 Leuven, Belgium.

However, several questions regarding which swallowing structures are essential, and what volume and dose constraints should be applied, remain to be answered.

Obviously, efficient swallowing is an extremely complex process, consisting of a series of coordinated events involving more than 30 pairs of muscles and 6 cranial nerves. Based on the physiology and anatomy of normal swallowing, a number of potential organs at risk for swallowing dysfunction have been identified. Correlating the dose to these structures with the presence of late dysphagia allows the definition of dose-response curves. However, it is not clear how the endpoint of dysphagia should be best described. Objective assessment is possible through invasive techniques such as videofluoroscopy with modified barium swallow or fiberoptic endoscopic evaluation of swallowing. There are also several validated questionnaires for subjective evaluation, such as the EORTC QLQ-HandN35 swallowing subscale, consisting of 4 questions regarding swallowing of liquid, swallowing of pureed food, swallowing of solid food, and aspiration when swallowing. Experience in the evaluation of xerostomia has indicated that patient-reported endpoints are preferable.

Despite the use of different dysphagia endpoints, different sets of potential organs at risk and different patient populations, results of published studies determining the critical structures for the prevention of swallowing complications are remarkably consistent. Apparently, both the mean dose to the pharyngeal constrictor muscles and the larynx, as well as the volume of those structures receiving 50 – 60 Gy, is significantly correlated with the occurrence of late dysphagia. These data imply that sparing these structures could prevent late dysphagia. However, no clear dose or volume constraints can yet be proposed, and currently, the best approach consists of keeping the radiation dose to these structures as low as possible. On the other hand, avoiding underdosing to the targets in the vicinity should remain the highest priority.

Introduction

Head and Neck Cancer

Head and neck cancer (HNC) is a broad term that encompasses all epithelial malignancies arising from the upper gastro-intestinal and airway tracts, thus including tumors originating from a wide variety of sub-sites such as the nasal cavity and paranasal sinuses, nasopharynx, oral cavity, oropharynx, larynx, hypopharynx, or salivary glands. It constitutes the fifth most common malignancy worldwide, representing about 6% of all cancers and yearly accounting for an estimated 47,560 new cases in the United States alone and at least 500,000 worldwide [1]. The overall majority of these epithelial malignancies are squamous cell carcinoma (SCC), for which the most important risk factors are tobacco and alcohol consumption [2 – 4]. Other risk factors include viral infection, occupational exposure, radiation, dietary factors, and genetic susceptibility [2, 4]. Interestingly, there is increasing evidence documenting human papillomavirus (HPV), mainly HPV type 16 and to a lesser extent type 18, as an important cause of specific subsets of head and neck cancer, perhaps establishing a particular entity [5, 6].

Treatment for HNC is highly complex, not only because of the variety of disease subsites, but also because of the intricate anatomy, with normal and tumoral structures often in close proximity, and the importance of preserving organ function. While radiotherapy (RT) and surgery remain the two main treatment options, systemic therapy has recently become an integral part of multidisciplinary treatment. The choice of modality depends upon patient factors, primary site, clinical stage, and resectability of the tumor [7].

Approximately 30% to 40% of patients present with early (stage I and II) disease. These patients can be effectively treated with either surgery or definitive radiotherapy. Both modalities result in similar rates of loco-regional control and survival, so the choice is usually based on the morbidity and functional outcome that can be expected [8].

However, more than half of patients present with loco-regionally advanced (stage III or IV) disease at diagnosis. Management of these patients requires aggressive and concerted measures, and remains a clinical challenge. Patients can be treated with complete surgical excision followed by post-operative (chemo-) radiotherapy or with primary (chemo-) radiotherapy. Until recently, 5-year survival rates were reported to be below 30% for patients with stage IV disease and 40% for all loco-regionally advanced tumors [9]. However, intensification of radiotherapy treatment using altered fractionation schedules and/or concomitant chemotherapy has resulted in significantly improved loco-regional control and survival rates.

An important randomized trial by the radiation therapy oncology group (RTOG), comparing 3 types of altered fractionation, showed a significant loco-regional control and survival benefit with both hyperfractionation and concomitant-boost RT, but not with accelerated fractionation [10]. This observation is consistent with the results of a large meta-analysis by Bourhis et al., showing an absolute survival benefit of 8% at 5 years for schedules with increased total dose, compared to only 2% for accelerated fractionation. The use of any type of altered fractionation schedule leads to an absolute survival benefit of 3.4% at 5 years [11]. Most altered fractionation schedules significantly increase acute toxicity, predominantly mucositis and dysphagia [12]. Late toxicity is generally not increased after modestly accelerated or hyperfractionated RT, although highly accelerated trials did show elevated late toxicity [12].

Similarly, clinical trials with the use of systemic chemotherapy (Cx) in HNC demonstrated successful anti-tumor activity [13]. Therefore, chemotherapy was increasingly added to primary radiotherapy, with most clinicians opting for a concurrent delivery of the two modalities. The rationale for this was that tumor cell clonogens could be sensitized to radiation by the concurrent delivery of Cx, thereby possibly enhancing loco-regional control. A large investigation from the meta-analysis of chemotherapy in head and neck cancer (MACH-NC) collaborative group, as well as its updates in 2004 and 2009, showed an absolute survival benefit of 6.5% at 5 years for concomitant chemoradiotherapy (CRT), making this approach the new standard of care [14 – 16]. The largest benefit was observed with platinum-based Cx, and no significant difference was seen between mono- or poly- chemotherapy [14 – 16]. Obviously, the sensitizing effect of Cx is not selective for tumor cells, and adjacent normal tissues within the radiation field are also subjected to more effective and thus more toxic RT. Consistently, CRT trials report an increased incidence of toxicities, with mucositis, dysphagia, and dermatitis being the most prominent.

Clearly, intensification of radiotherapy treatment for locally advanced head and neck cancer through the use of altered fractionation schedules and/or concomitant chemotherapy has resulted in significantly improved loco-regional control and survival rates. However, concomitant chemotherapy in particular is associated with high rates of early and late swallowing problems [17 – 19]. For example, in an analysis of HNC patients treated with or without concomitant chemotherapy, we observed a significantly higher incidence of grade 3 dysphagia (82.2% vs. 47.9%, p < 0.0001) in the chemoradiotherapy group [20]. At the moment, no further treatment intensification appears possible without effective techniques to prevent serious late complications, and especially late dysphagia [21].

Radiotherapy

The introduction of conformal radiotherapy with three-dimensional (3D) treatment planning on computed tomography (CT) scans signified a first major improvement over conventional two-dimensional (2D) radiotherapy, where the treatment portals are based on a radiographic simulation film. Forward treatment planning is employed for both 2D-RT and 3D-RT, which essentially consists of the radiation oncologist designing the RT fields and the radiation physicist generating an optimized dose distribution. In contrast, inverse treatment planning is employed with intensity-modulated radiotherapy (IMRT) and consists of identifying the target volumes and organs at risk (OAR) on the planning CT. The dose to the tumor is specified, as well as the maximum acceptable doses to adjacent normal structures, and the physicist uses that information to produce the optimal plan, i.e. one that ensures target coverage by the prescribed radiation dose while reducing doses to the organs at risk.

The basic principle behind IMRT is the use of intensity-modulated beams, i.e. beams with several dose intensity levels, essentially adding an additional dimension to the treatment planning. Usually, 5 to 7 non-opposing, co-planar beams are combined to "sculpt" the high-dose areas around the target volumes, with steep dose fall-off immediately outside these regions, thus allowing highly conformal radiation dose delivery. The most popular way to perform spatial modulation of beam intensity is through the use of a multileaf collimator (MLC), although other solutions exist. An MLC consists of a high number (up to 120) of individual leaves that can move independently of each other. Step-and-shoot IMRT occurs when the leaves move when the beam is off, but do not move when the beam is on. Another solution is dynamic IMRT, whereby the leaves move continuously at various speed during irradiation.

Static beam IMRT has evolved to rotational IMRT offering even a more conform dose distribution. There are basically two major ways to perform rotational radiotherapy. On the one hand, there are the volumetric modulated arc therapy (VMAT) systems, which treat the whole tumour volume at once during the gantry rotation while modifying the dose rate, the gantry speed, and the shape of the beam. On the other hand, there are the specifically designed systems for IMRT, with integrated CT-scan to combine high quality IMRT with high precision image guided radiotherapy (IGRT), for example Helical Tomotherapy.

The major advantage of IMRT is a more conformal dose distribution with steep dose gradients between the target volumes and the critical OAR, which should result in decreased toxicity and could possibly allow for the delivery of a higher radiation dose to the tumor (i.e. dose-escalation), in an effort to improve loco-regional control [22 – 24]. Since IMRT delivers highly conformal dose distributions to target volumes of almost any shape, appropriate selection and accurate delineation of the target volumes and the avoidable organs are of critical importance [25]. Recommendation guidelines for the selection of the clinical target volume for both the primary tumors and neck nodal areas have been produced [26 – 29]. Regarding the sparing of organs at risk, some suggestions were recently made [30, 31].

Reducing Toxicity

The organs at risk in the head and neck region include the spinal cord, brainstem, salivary glands, swallowing structures, and mandible. For nasopharynx cancer, the optic nerves, chiasm, and temporal lobes of the brain are also at risk. Exceeding the tolerances of these structures can lead to cord or brainstem dysfunction, xerostomia, dysphagia, osteoradionecrosis, blindness, or brain necrosis. Thus, organ-sparing radiotherapy requires the appropriate selection and accurate delineation of multiple avoidance structures. However, the construction of dose-response curves, allowing the definition of reliable radiation dose constraints below which a complication is unlikely to occur, is a complicated process. Most available data are based on expert opinion or retrospective analyses, often insufficiently correcting for confounding clinical factors, and using different endpoints to define a complication in disparate patient populations, making the proposal of definitive conclusions difficult.

Moreover, there is increasing concern that inappropriate sparing of normal tissue, perhaps due to an overemphasis on toxicity prevention rather than tumor eradication in recent literature, could lead to avoidable marginal recurrences [32, 33]. Obviously, the shielding of clinically negative, at-risk regions from elective radiation to prevent damage to healthy tissue should be approached with extreme care: adequate selection of patients is of crucial importance and loco-regional recurrences need to be carefully evaluated and reported [25].

Xerostomia is usually considered to be the most prominent complication after radiotherapy for head and neck cancer. Radiation-induced damage to the salivary glands alters the volume, consistency, and pH of secreted saliva. Saliva changes from thin secretions with a neutral pH to thick and tenacious secretions with increased acidity. Patients suffer from oral discomfort or pain, find it difficult to speak, chew or swallow, and run an increased risk of dental caries or oral infection. Ultimately, this can lead to decreased nutritional intake and weight loss. Radiation-induced xerostomia not only significantly reduces the quality of life of potentially cured patients, but also poses a major new health problem for them [34].

Swallowing dysfunction after radiotherapy is correlated with compromised quality of life (QoL), and can lead to life-threatening complications such as aspiration pneumonia [17 – 19, 35]. Because the risk of radiation-induced dysphagia is associated with the use of altered fractionation schedules and especially concomitant chemotherapy, its incidence has considerably increased in recent years [17 – 20]. Currently, the impact of late dysphagia on health-related QoL after radiotherapy is at least as important as that of permanent xerostomia [36]. Moreover, xerostomia can now be successfully avoided in a large subset of patients, while no comparable advances were made regarding the prevention of dysphagia. These observations have prompted something of a shift of focus towards the prevention of swallowing problems, and have led some to suggest that late dysphagia, rather than xerostomia, is the dose-limiting toxicity of chemoradiotherapy and therefore constitutes the main obstacle towards further treatment intensification [21, 37]. It is to be expected that, similar to salivary gland-sparing radiotherapy, limiting the radiation dose to the critical swallowing structures will reduce the incidence and severity of radiation-induced dysphagia [38]. However, several questions regarding which swallowing structures are essential, and what volume and dose constraints should be applied, remain to be answered.

Radiation-Induced Dysphagia

(Patho-) Physiology of Swallowing

Obviously, efficient swallowing is an extremely complex process, consisting of a series of coordinated events involving more than 30 pairs of muscles and 6 cranial nerves [39]. Swallowing consists of three phases (oral (preparatory), pharyngeal, and esophageal), with the voluntary oral preparatory and oral phases followed by an involuntary reflex that must be triggered. This process implies a rapid and precise coordination between sensory input and motor function. Swallowing involves controlling the food in the mouth, largely with the oral part of the tongue, to enable tasting and chewing to occur. The oral tongue moves the food onto the teeth to crush the food, collects the food from around the mouth after chewing, brings it together to form a bolus, and propels it backward out of the mouth. Thereafter, the pharyngeal stage of swallowing is triggered and a number of necessary motor activities occur: (1) hyoid movement, (2) closure of the entrance to the nose, the velopharyngeal port, by elevation of the soft palate to prevent food from entering the nose, (3) closure of the airway to prevent food from entering the lungs, (4) opening of the upper esophageal sphincter by relaxation of the cricopharyngeal muscles and by movement of the larynx anteriorly and superiorly to enable the bolus to pass into the esophagus, (5) epiglottic inversion, and (6) pharyngeal contraction to push the food through the pharynx and the esophagus. All these actions must be appropriately coordinated for the swallow to be safe and efficient.

Post-radiotherapy dysphagia is due to neuromuscular fibrosis and radiation-induced edema, leading to abnormal motility of deglutition muscles such as impaired pharyngeal contraction and laryngeal elevation [39]. Probably, sensory changes in the oral cavity and the pharynx also play a role by changing the patient's perception of swallowing. There are hypotheses that RT can have an effect on innervation of the larynx and pharynx, causing loss of laryngeal sensation, motor function, and normal peristalsis. Obviously, xerostomia after RT due to the inclusion of salivary glands in the radiation field contributes to swallowing problems [34].

Incidence and Impact

The incidence and severity of post-RT dysphagia is dependent on several factors: total radiation dose, fraction size, fractionation schedule, target volumes, interfraction interval, treatment techniques, use of concomitant chemotherapy, smoking during and after RT, percutaneous endoscopic gastrostomy (PEG) tube feeding or prolonged (> 1 − 2 weeks) nil per os, depression, and poor mental health [40, 41]. The meta-analysis of Machtay et al. showed that older age, advanced tumor stage, larynx/hypopharynx primary site, and neck dissection after concomitant CRT are the main clinical risk factors for severe late toxicity [42]. Langendijk and colleagues recently developed a predictive model for swallowing dysfunction after curative RT for head and neck cancer (the total dysphagia risk score or TDRS). They observed that T3-4 T-classification, bilateral neck irradiation, weight loss prior to RT, oropharyngeal and nasopharyngeal tumors, accelerated radiotherapy and concomitant chemotherapy were independent prognostic factors for swallowing disorders. Based on the presence or absence of these clinical factors, patients can be classified into three risk groups (low, intermediate or high risk), correlating with the onset of acute dysphagia and late swallowing dysfunction [43]. This risk score was recently validated by researchers from a different group [44]. An average rate of 50% dysphagia after chemoradiotherapy for advanced HNC is reported [45]. However, it should be noted that the incidence of dysphagia is probably underreported in trials because clinical judgment often underestimates the severity of swallowing problems [17 – 19].

Little is known about the evolution of swallowing problems after CRT, but dysphagia and aspiration can begin or significantly worsen years after treatment. This is probably due to submucosal effects such as fibrosis and vascular and nerve (sensory and motor) injury. Nguyen et al. reported that the severity of dysphagia decreased in 32%, remained unchanged in 48%, and worsened in 20% of patients at one year or more following RT [46]. Goguen et al. described dysphagia as slowly but only partly resolving after 6–12 months following CRT for advanced HNC [47]. However, in another study on nasopharyngeal cancer patients treated with RT, a continuous deterioration of swallowing function over time was seen [48].

Swallowing dysfunction has a clear negative impact on the global quality of life of HNC patients. Dysphagia leads to longer eating times, inability to eat different types of food, and fear or inability to eat in public, which in turn results in social isolation and depression [49]. Obviously, prolonged unnatural feeding may induce major psychological distress because it causes discomfort and distorts the patient's self-image. Nguyen et al. found that the severity of dysphagia correlates with compromised QoL, anxiety, and depression [35]. Langendijk et al. clearly showed that the effect of late radiation-induced toxicity, particularly on swallowing function and salivary gland function, has a significant impact on the more general dimensions of health-related (HR) QoL, such as physical, social, and mental health [36]. They further described that the impact of radiation-induced swallowing dysfunction is greatest in the first 12 months after completion of RT and gradually decreases at 18 and 24 months [36]. Clearly, dysphagia has a devastating effect on patient daily life.

Scoring Dysphagia

Based on the physiology and anatomy of normal swallowing, a number of potential organs at risk for swallowing dysfunction can be identified. Correlating the radiation dose to these structures with the presence of late dysphagia could allow the definition of dose-response curves. However, it is not clear how the endpoint of dysphagia should be best described. Objective assessment is possible through invasive techniques such as videofluoroscopy with modified barium swallow (VF-MBS) or fiberoptic endoscopic evaluation of swallowing (FEES).

Videofluoroscopy, developed by Logemann, is a validated standard method that allows viewing and recording of the structures and dynamics of the swallowing process [50]. The whole assessment focuses on bolus manipulation, bolus control, and bolus passage including cohesion, motility, and timing. The findings of each patient are scored using the swallowing performance scale (SPS). This is a validated and accurate assessment of dysphagia severity by combining clinical and radiographic information. The severity of dysphagia is graded on a scale of 1–7 [51].

A second objective tool to evaluate swallowing dysfunction is functional endoscopic evaluation of swallowing [52]. It visualizes the pharynx from above by placing an endoscopic tube, without anesthesia, transnasally such that the end of the tube hangs over the end of the soft palate. The anatomy and function of the soft palate, tongue base, pharynx, and larynx are assessed during speech, spontaneous movements, dry swallowing, and swallowing of various consistencies of liquid and food. Sensitivity of the pharynx is assessed by light touch with the tip of the endoscope. Premature leakage of food or fluid from the mouth into the pharynx before a voluntary swallow can be assessed. Residue in vallecula epiglottica, aryepiglottic region, and piriform sinus can be assessed together with laryngeal penetration and aspiration.

Several validated questionnaires for subjective evaluation also exist, such as the EORTC QLQ-HandN35 swallowing subscale (HNSW), consisting of 4 questions regarding swallowing of liquid, swallowing of pureed food, swallowing of solid food, and aspiration when swallowing; the performance status scale (PSS) of List, with the functions eating in public and normalcy of diet; and the MD Anderson dysphagia inventory (MDADI), consisting of 20 questions with global, emotional, functional, and physical subscales [53 – 56]. As for xerostomia, objective evaluation of swallowing is not always representative of patient-reported symptoms [57]. However, experience in the evaluation of xerostomia has indicated that patient-reported endpoints are preferable [34, 58].

Prevention of Radiation-Induced Dysphagia

Dysphagia and Aspiration-Related Structures (DARS)

Clinical trials to analyze the relationship between irradiated structures and dysphagia have produced consistent data regarding the crucial structures associated with swallowing dysfunctions. Based on a literature search, anatomic text books and radiological data, 8 potential "swallowing structures" were identified: 1) superior pharyngeal constrictor (SPC) muscle; 2) middle pharyngeal constrictor (MPC) muscle; 3) inferior pharyngeal constrictor (IPC) muscle; 4) base of tongue (BOT); 5) supraglottic larynx (SGL); 6) glottic larynx (GL); 7) upper esophageal sphincter (UES), including the cricopharyngeus muscle; 8) esophagus (ES) [30, 38, 39]. Definitions of the swallowing OAR are provided in Table 1.

Eisbruch et al. were the first to suggest both the pharyngeal constrictor muscles and the larynx as the critical organs at risk for late dysphagia [59]. When tested in a prospective study using IMRT, both the mean dose to the pharyngeal constrictor muscles (especially the SPC muscle) and the larynx, as well as the volume of those structures receiving $\geq$ 50 Gy (V50), appeared to be the most significant predictors [60]. Levendag et al. observed a significant correlation between the presence of late dysphagia and the mean dose to the superior and middle pharyngeal constrictor muscles [61]. These data were further supported in two other studies by the same group [62, 63]. Jensen et al. found a correlation between late dysphagia and the mean dose to the larynx, as well as the volume of the larynx receiving $\geq$ 60 Gy (V60) [64]. A study by Caglar et al. also found the mean dose to the inferior pharyngeal constrictor muscle and the larynx, as well as the V50 of those structures, to correlate with aspiration [65]. In our own study, the mean dose to the middle and inferior pharyngeal constrictor muscles and supraglottic larynx, as well as the partial volume of these structures receiving $\geq$ 50 Gy, significantly correlated with late dysphagia [66]. Recently, Caudell and colleagues found that doses to the larynx and (inferior) pharyngeal constrictors predicted long-term swallowing complications, whether PEG tube dependence at 12 months, aspiration on VF-MBS or pharyngoesophageal stricture requiring dilation, even when controlled for other clinical factors [67].

Table 1. Proposed delineation guidelines for the swallowing structures

OAR	Superior border	Inferior border	Anterior border	Posterior border
1. Superior pharyngeal constrictor muscle	caudal tip of the pterygoid plates (hamulus)	upper edge of hyoid bone	widest diameter of rhinopharynx, base of tongue, hyoid bone and larynx	cervical vertebra or pre-vertebral muscles
2. Middle pharyngeal constrictor muscle	upper edge of hyoid bone	lower edge of hyoid bone		
3. Inferior pharyngeal constrictor muscle	lower edge of hyoid bone	lower edge of cricoid cartilage		
4. Base of tongue	below soft palate (uvula)	upper edge of hyoid bone	posterior third of the tongue	
5. Supraglottic larynx (lumen excluded)	top of the piriform sinus and aryepiglottic fold	upper edge of the cricoid cartilage	anterior tip of the thyroid cartilage	cornu of the thyroid cartilage
6. Glottic larynx (lumen excluded)	at the level of the cricoid cartilage			
7. Upper esophageal sphincter including m. cricopharyngeus	lower edge of cricoid cartilage	upper edge of trachea	subglottic larynx	cervical vertebra
8. Esophagus	upper edge of trachea	first 2 cm	trachea	cervical vertebra

Table 2. Overview of studies evaluating critical structures for late dysphagia

Study	No.	Site	Dosimetric parameter							End-point
			mean PC	mean Larynx	mean ES	V50 PC	V60 PC	V50 Larynx	V60 Larynx	
Feng, 2007 [60]	36	OP/NP	0.008	0.032	NS	0.008	0.006	0.016	NS	VF
Levendag, 2007 [61]	56	OP	0.02	-	NS	-	-	-	-	HNSW
Teguh, 2008 [62]	81	OP/NP	0.01	-	NS	-	-	-	-	HNSW
Teguh, 2008 [63]	20	OP	0.04	-	NS	-	-	-	-	FEES
Jensen, 2007 [64]	25	Pharynx	NS	0.048	NS	NS	NS	NS	0.035	HNSW
Caglar, 2008 [65]	96	all	0.007	0.003	NS	0.05	NS	0.04	NS	VF
Dirix, 2009 [66]	53	all	0.02	0.04	NS	0.04	NS	0.08	NS	HNSW
Caudell, 2010 [67]	83	all	NS	0.002	NS	NS	0.02	NS	<0.001	VF

Abbreviations: No.: number of patients included in the analysis; OP: oropharynx; NP: nasopharynx; PC: pharyngeal constrictor muscles; ES: esophagus; VF: videofluoroscopy; HNSW: EORTC QLQ-HandN35 swallowing symptom score; FEES: fiberoptic endoscopic evaluation of swallowing.

Interestingly, a recent study found that perfusion changes in the pharyngeal constrictor muscles on CT perfusion (CTP) imaging during the second week of RT may predict for the severity of late dysphagia. The CTP parameters at week 2 of RT demonstrated an increase in mean PC blood flow of 161.9% vs. 12.3% (p = 0.007) and an increase in mean PC blood volume of 96.6% vs. 8.7% (p = 0.039) in patients with 6-month post-RT grade 3 dysphagia and grade 0-2 dysphagia, respectively [68]. On multivariate analysis, when adjusting for smoking history, tumor volume, and baseline dysphagia status, an increase in blood flow in the second week of RT was significantly predictive for grade 3 dysphagia at 3 and 6 months after RT (p < 0.05). These findings further emphasize the importance of the pharyngeal constrictor muscles in the onset of late swallowing problems.

DARS Dose Constraints?

So despite the use of different dysphagia endpoints, sets of potential organs at risk and patient populations, results of published studies determining the critical structures for the prevention of swallowing complications are remarkably consistent (Table 2). Apparently, both the mean dose to the pharyngeal constrictor muscles and the larynx, as well as the volume of those structures receiving 50 – 60 Gy, is significantly correlated with the occurrence of late dysphagia [60 – 67]. These data imply that sparing these structures could prevent late dysphagia. A dose–risk ratio, based on retrospective analysis, has even been suggested by some investigators. Levendag et al. for instance reported a 19% increase in the probability of dysphagia with every additional 10 Gy to the superior and middle constrictor muscles [61]. Li et al. suggested that to reduce the risk of prolonged PEG tube use, the dose constraints should be a mean dose of <55 Gy to the inferior constrictor muscle, and a maximum dose of <60 Gy to the cricopharyngeal inlet [69]. Obviously, all the limitations of a retrospective analysis apply to these data, and the current evidence is not strong enough to suggest clear volume or dose constraints.

Prospective, longitudinal studies including baseline evaluation with predetermined follow-up assessment at different time points are needed to better understand the relationship between dose or volume and swallowing outcomes. Feng et al. demonstrated a significant correlation between aspirations on videofluoroscopy and the mean doses to the pharyngeal constrictor muscles and the glottic and supraglottic larynx, as well as the partial volumes of these structures receiving 50–65 Gy [60]. A prospective trial was conducted by the same authors using these dose–volume parameters as initial IMRT optimization goals, and the results suggested that IMRT with concurrent chemotherapy planned to reduce dysphagia can be performed safely for oropharyngeal cancer [70]. At one year after treatment, average patient-reported, observer-rated, and objective measures of swallowing were only slightly worse than pretherapy measures, representing potential improvement compared with previous studies [70]. Therefore, the routine IMRT practice at the University of Michigan is to keep the mean dose to the non-involved pharyngeal constrictor muscles and glottic and supraglottic larynx ≤50 Gy [31].

However, no clear dose or volume constraints can yet be proposed, and currently, the best approach consists of keeping the radiation dose to these structures as low as possible. However, avoiding underdosing to the targets in the vicinity should retain the highest priority.

It is also to be expected that more selective delineation of the elective nodal volume will facilitate the successful sparing of the swallowing structures. Of particular importance is the delineation of the retropharyngeal (RP) lymph nodes, located between the pharyngeal constrictor muscles and the prevertebral fascia, from the base of skull to the caudal border of C2. The medial RP nodes, located near the midline and anterior to the prevertebral musculature, are only very rarely involved as metastatic sites [71, 72]. Therefore, their exclusion from the elective target volume could considerably contribute to the sparing of the pharyngeal constrictor muscles [30, 31, 38].

Conclusion

To prevent late dysphagia, the best approach consists of reducing the doses to the pharyngeal constrictor muscles and the larynx as much as possible, although avoiding target underdosing remains the highest priority. It is to be expected that prospective collection of dosimetric data, adequately correcting for confounding clinical parameters, along with the corresponding functional outcomes, preferably based on patient-reported or quality of life endpoints, will allow determining more precise dose-response curves.

References

[1] Jemal A., Siegel R., Ward E., et al. Cancer statistics, 2009. CA *Cancer J. Clin.* 2009; 59: 225 – 249.

[2] Spitz M.R. Epidemiology and risk factors for head and neck cancer. *Semin. Oncol.* 1994; 21: 281 – 288.

[3] Lewin F., Norell S.E., Johansson H., et al. Smoking tobacco, oral snuff and alcohol in the etiology of squamous cell carcinoma of the head and neck: a population-based case-referent study in Sweden. *Cancer* 1998; 82: 1367 – 1375.

[4] Argiris A., Eng C. Epidemiology, staging, and screening of head and neck cancer. *Cancer Treat Res* 2003; 114: 15 – 60.

[5] Mork J., Lie K., Glattre E., et al. Human papilloma virus infection as a risk factor for squamous cell carcinoma of the head and neck. *N Engl J Med* 2001; 344: 1125 – 1131.

[6] D'Souza G., Kreimer A.R., Viscidi R., et al. Case-control study of human papillomavirus and oropharyngeal cancer. *N Engl J Med* 2007; 356: 1944 – 1956.

[7] Argiris A., Karamouzis M.V., Raben D., Ferris R.L. Head and neck cancer. *Lancet* 2008; 371: 1695 – 1709.

[8] Forastiere A.A., Koch W., Trotti A., Sidransky D. Head and neck cancer. Medical progress. *N Engl J Med* 2001; 345: 1890 – 1900.

[9] Seiwert T.Y., Cohen E.E.W. State-of-the-art management of locally advanced head and neck cancer. *Br J Cancer* 2005; 92: 1341 – 1348.

[10] Fu K.K., Pajak T.F., Trotti A., et al. A Radiation Therapy Oncology Group (RTOG) phase III randomized study to compare hyperfractionation and two variants of accelerated fractionation to standard fractionation therapy for head and neck squamous cell carcinomas: first report of RTOG 90-03. *Int J Radiat Oncol Biol Phys* 2000; 48: 7 – 16.

[11] Bourhis J., Overgaard J., Audry H., et al. Hyperfractionated or accelerated radiotherapy in head and neck cancer: a meta-analysis. *Lancet* 2006; 368: 843 – 584.

[12] Nguyen L.N., Ang K.K. Radiotherapy for cancer of the head and neck: altered fractionation regimens. *Lancet Oncol* 2002; 3: 693 – 701.

[13] Vermorken J.B. Medical treatment in head and neck cancer. *Ann Oncol* 2005; 16: 258 – 264.

[14] Pignon J.P., Bourhis J., Domenge C., Designe L. on behalf of the MACH-NC Collaborative Group. Chemotherapy added to locoregional

treatment for head and neck squamous-cell carcinoma: three meta-analyses of updated individual data. *Lancet* 2000; 355: 949 – 955.

[15] Bourhis J., Amand C., Pignon J.P. on behalf of the MACH-NC Collaborative Group. Update of the MACH-NC (meta-analysis of chemotherapy in head and neck cancer) database focused on concomitant chemoradiotherapy. *J Clin Oncol* 2004; 22: S5505.

[16] Pignon J.P., le Maître A., Maillard E., Bourhis J. on behalf of the MACH-NC Collaborative Group. Meta-analysis of chemotherapy in head and neck cancer (MACH-NC): an update on 93 randomised trials and 17,346 patients. *Radiother Oncol* 2009; 92: 4 – 14.

[17] Lazarus C.L., Logemann J.A., Pauloski B.R., et al. Swallowing disorders in head and neck cancer patients treated with radiotherapy and adjuvant chemotherapy. *Laryngoscope* 1996; 106: 1157 – 1166.

[18] Eisbruch A., Lyden T., Bradford C.R., et al. Objective assessment of swallowing dysfunction and aspiration after radiation concurrent with chemotherapy for head-and-neck cancer. *Int J Radiation Oncology Biol Phys* 2002; 53: 23 – 28.

[19] Nguyen N.P., Moltz C.C., Frank C.C., et al. Dysphagia following chemoradiation for locally advanced head and neck cancer. *Ann Oncol* 2004; 15: 383 – 388.

[20] Nuyts S., Dirix P., Clement P.M.J., et al. Impact of adding concomitant chemotherapy to hyperfractionated accelerated radiotherapy for advanced head and neck squamous cell carcinoma. *Int J Radiat Oncol Biol Phys* 2009, 73: 1088 – 1095.

[21] Robbins K.T. Barriers to winning the battle with head and neck cancer. *Int J Radiation Oncology Biol Phys* 2002; 53: 4 – 5.

[22] Veldeman L., Madani I., Hulstaert F., et al. Evidence behind use of intensity-modulated radiotherapy: a systematic review of comparative clinical studies. *Lancet Oncol* 2008; 9: 367 – 375.

[23] Dirix P., Vanstraelen B., Jorissen M., Vander Poorten V., Nuyts S. Intensity-modulated radiotherapy for sinonasal cancer: improved outcome compared to conventional radiotherapy. *Int J Radiat Oncol Biol Phys* 2010; 78: 998 – 1004.

[24] Dirix P., Nuyts S. Value of intensity-modulated radiotherapy in stage IV head and neck squamous cell carcinoma. *Int J Radiat Oncol Biol Phys* 2010; 78: 1373 – 1380.

[25] Harari P.M. Beware the swing and a miss: baseball precautions for conformal radiotherapy. *Int J Radiat Oncol Biol Phys* 2008; 70: 657 – 659.

[26] Chao K.S.C., Wippold F.J., Ozyigit G., et al. Determination and delineation of nodal target volumes for head-and-neck cancer based on patterns of failure in patients receiving definitive and postoperative IMRT. *Int J Radiat Oncol Biol Phys* 2002; 53: 1174 – 1184.

[27] Eisbruch A., Foote R.L., O'Sullivan B., et al. Intensity-modulated radiation therapy for head and neck cancer: emphasis on the selection and delineation of the targets. *Semin Radiat Oncol* 2002; 12: 238 – 249.

[28] Grégoire V., Levendag P., Ang K.K., et al. CT-based delineation of lymph node levels and related CTVs in the node-negative neck: DAHANCA, EORTC, GORTEC, NCIC, RTOG consensus guidelines. *Radiother Oncol* 2003; 69: 227 – 236.

[29] Grégoire V., Eisbruch A., Hamoir M., Levendag P. Proposal for the delineation of the nodal CTV in the node-positive and the post-operative neck. *Radiother Oncol* 2006; 79: 15 – 20.

[30] Dirix P., Nuyts S. Evidence-based organ-sparing radiotherapy in head and neck cancer. *Lancet Oncol* 2010; 11(1): 85 – 91.

[31] Wang X., Hu C., Eisbruch A. Organ-sparing radiation therapy for head and neck cancer. Nat Rev Clin Oncol 2011; Jul 26 [Epub ahead of print].

[32] Cannon D.M., Lee N.Y. Recurrence in region of spared parotid gland after definitive intensity-modulated radiotherapy for head and neck cancer. *Int J Radiat Oncol Biol Phys* 2008; 70: 660 – 665.

[33] Mendenhall W.M., Mancuso A.A. Radiotherapy for head and neck cancer – is the "next level" down? *Int J Radiat Oncol Biol Phys* 2009; 73: 645 – 646.

[34] Dirix P., Nuyts S., Van den Bogaert W. Radiation-induced xerostomia in patients with head and neck cancer: a literature review. *Cancer* 2006; 107: 2525 – 2534.

[35] Nguyen N.P., Frank C., Moltz C.C., et al. Impact of dysphagia on quality of life after treatment of head-and-neck cancer. *Int J Radiat Oncol Biol Phys* 2005; 61: 772 – 778.

[36] Langendijk J.A., Doornaert P., Verdonck-de Leeuw I.M., et al. Impact of late treatment-related toxicity on quality of life among patients with head and neck cancer treated with radiotherapy. *J Clin Oncol* 2008; 26: 3770 – 3776.

[37] Eisbruch A. Dysphagia and aspiration following chemo-irradiation of head and neck cancer: major obstacles to intensification of therapy. *Ann Oncol* 2004; 15: 363 – 364.

[38] Rosenthal D.I., Lewin J.S., Eisbruch A. Prevention and treatment of dysphagia and aspiration after chemoradiation for head and neck cancer. *J Clin Oncol* 2006; 24: 2636 – 2643.

[39] Platteaux N., Dirix P., Dejaeger E., Nuyts S. Dysphagia in head and neck cancer patients treated with chemoradiotherapy. *Dysphagia* 2010; 25: 139 – 152.

[40] Caudell J.J., Schaner P.E., Meredith R.F., et al. Factors associated with long-term dysphagia after definitive radiotherapy for locally advanced head-and-neck cancer. *Int. J. Radiat. Oncol. Biol. Phys.* 2009; 73: 410 – 415.

[41] Koiwai K., Shikama N., Sasaki S., et al. Risk factors for severe dysphagia after concurrent chemoradiotherapy for head and neck cancers. *Jpn J Clin Oncol* 2009; 37: 413 – 417.

[42] Machtay M., Moughan J., Trotti A., et al. Factors associated with severe late toxicity after concurrent chemoradiation for locally advanced head and neck cancer: an RTOG analysis. *J Clin Oncol* 2008; 26: 3582 – 3589.

[43] Langendijk J.A., Doornaert P., Rietveld D.H.F., et al. A predictive model for swallowing dysfunction after curative radiotherapy in head and neck cancer. *Radiother Oncol* 2009; 90: 189 – 195.

[44] Koiwai K., Shikama N., Sasaki S., et al. Validation of the total dysphagia risk score (TDRS) as a predictive measure for acute swallowing dysfunction induced by chemoradiotherapy for head and neck cancers. *Radiother Oncol* 2010; 97: 132 – 135.

[45] Nguyen N.P., Sallah S., Karlsson U., Antoine J.E. Combined chemotherapy and radiation therapy for head and neck malignancies: quality of life issues. *Cancer* 2002; 94: 1131 – 1141.

[46] Nguyen N.P., Moltz C.C., Frank C., et al. Evolution of chronic dysphagia following treatment for head and neck cancer. *Oral Oncol* 2006; 42: 374 – 380.

[47] Goguen L.A., Posner M.R., Norris C.M., et al. Dysphagia after sequential chemoradiation therapy for advanced head and neck cancer. *Otolaryngol Head Neck Surg* 2006; 134: 916 – 922.

[48] Chang Y.C., Chen S.Y., Lui L.T., et al. Dysphagia in patients with nasopharyngeal cancer after radiation therapy: a videofluoroscopic swallowing study. *Dysphagia* 2003; 18: 135 – 143.

[49] Gillespie M.B., Brodsky M.B., Day T.A., Lee F.S., Martin-Harris B. Swallowing-related quality of life after head and neck cancer treatment. *Laryngoscope* 2004; 114: 1362 – 1367.

[50] Logemann JA. *Evaluation, treatment of swallowing disorders.* San Diego, CA: College Hill Press; 1983. p. 3–70.

[51] Logemann JA. *Manual for the videofluorographic study of swallowing.* San Diego, CA: College Hill Press; 1986.

[52] Bastian R.W. Videoendoscopic evaluation of patients with dysphagia: an adjunct to the modified barium swallow. *Otolaryngol Head Neck Surg* 1991; 104: 339 – 350.

[53] Bjordal K, de Graeff A, Fayers PM, Hammerlid E, van Pottelsberghe C, Curran D, et al. A 12 country field study of the EORTC QLQ-C3.0 (version 30) and the head and neck cancer specific module (EORTC QLQ-HandN35) in head and neck patients. EORTC Quality of Life Group. *Eur J Cancer.* 2000;36(14):1796–807.

[54] Sherman AC, Simonton S, Adams DC, Vural E, Owens B, Hanna E. Assessing quality of life in patients with head and neck cancer: cross-validation of the European Organization for Research and Treatment of Cancer (EORTC) Quality of Life Head and Neck module (QLQ-HandN35). *Arch Otolaryngol Head Neck Surg.* 2000;126(4):459–67.

[55] List MA, D'Antonio LL, Cella DF, Siston A, Mumby P, Haraf D, et al. The Performance Status Scale for Head and Neck Cancer Patients and the Functional Assessment of Cancer Therapy-Head and Neck Scale A study of utility and validity. *Cancer.* 1996;77(11):2294–301.

[56] Chen AY, Frankowski R, Bishop-Leone J, Hebert T, Leyk S, Lewin J, et al. The development and validation of a dysphagia-specific quality-of-life questionnaire for patients with head and neck cancer: the M. D. Anderson dysphagia inventory. *Arch Otolaryngol Head Neck Surg.* 2001;127(7):870–6.

[57] Jensen K., Jensen A.B., Grau C. The relationship between observer-based toxicity scoring and patient assessed symptom severity after treatment for head and neck cancer. A correlative cross-sectional study of the DAHANCA toxicity scoring system and the EORTC quality of life questionnaires. *Radiother Oncol* 2006; 78: 298 – 305.

[58] Meirovitz A., Murdoch-Kinch C.A., Schipper M., Pan C., Eisbruch A. Grading xerostomia by physicians or by patients after intensity-modulated radiotherapy of head-and-neck cancer. *Int J Radiation Oncology Biol Phys* 2006; 66: 445 – 453.

[59] Eisbruch A., Schwartz M., Rasch C., et al. Dysphagia and aspiration after chemoradiotherapy for head and neck cancer: which anatomic structures are affected and can they be spared by IMRT? *Int J Radiation Oncology Biol Phys* 2004; 60: 1425 – 1439.

[60] Feng F.Y., Kim H.M., Lyden T.H., et al. Intensity-modulated radiotherapy of head and neck cancer aiming to reduce dysphagia: early-dose effect relationships for the swallowing structures. *Int J Radiation Oncology Biol Phys* 2007; 68: 1289 – 1298.

[61] Levendag P.C., Teguh D.N., Voet P., et al. Dysphagia disorders in patients with cancer of the oropharynx are significantly affected by the radiation therapy dose to the superior and middle constrictor muscle: a dose-effect relationship. *Radiother Oncol* 2007; 85: 64 – 73.

[62] Teguh D.N., Levendag P.C., Noever I., et al. Treatment techniques and site considerations regarding dysphagia-related quality of life in cancer of the oropharynx and nasopharynx. *Int J Radiat Oncol Biol Phys* 2008; 72: 1119 – 1127.

[63] Teguh D.N., Levendag P.C., Sewnaik A., et al. Results of fiberoptic endoscopic evaluation of swallowing vs. radiation dose in the swallowing muscles after radiotherapy of cancer in the oropharynx. *Radiother Oncol* 2008; 89: 57 – 64.

[64] Jensen K., Lambertsen K., Grau C. Late swallowing dysfunction and dysphagia after radiotherapy for pharynx cancer: frequency, intensity and correlation with dose and volume parameters. *Radiother Oncol* 2007; 85: 74 – 82.

[65] Caglar H.B., Tishler R.B., Othus M., et al. Dose to larynx predicts for swallowing complications after intensity-modulated radiotherapy. Int J *Radiation Oncology Biol Phys* 2008; 72: 1110 – 1118.

[66] Dirix P., Abbeel S., Vanstraelen B., Hermans R., Nuyts S. Dysphagia after chemoradiotherapy for head and neck squamous cell carcinoma: dose-effect relationships for the swallowing structures. *Int J Radiat Oncol Biol Phys* 2009; 75: 385 – 392.

[67] Caudell J.J., Schaner P.E., Desmond R.A., et al. Dosimetric factors associated with long-term dysphagia after radiotherapy for squamous cell carcinoma of the head and neck. *Int J Radiat Oncol Biol Phys* 2009; 76: 403 – 409.

[68] Truong M.T., Lee R., Saito N., et al. Correlating CT perfusion changes in the pharyngeal constrictor muscles during head-and-neck radiotherapy to dysphagia outcome. *Int J Radiat Oncol Biol Phys* 2011; Jun 11 [Epub ahead of print].

[69] Li B., Li D., Lau D. H., et al. Clinical-dosimetric analysis of measures of dysphagia including gastrostomy-tube dependence among head and neck cancer patients treated definitively by intensity-modulated radiotherapy with concurrent chemotherapy. *Radiat Oncol* 2009; 4: 52.

[70] Feng F.Y., Kim H.M., Lyde T. H., et al. Intensity-modulated chemoradiotherapy aiming to reduce dysphagia in patients with oropharyngeal cancer: clinical and functional results. *J Clin Oncol* 2010; 28: 2732 – 2738.

[71] Bussels B., Hermans R., Reijnders A., Dirix P., Nuyts S., Van den Bogaert W. Retropharyngeal nodes in squamous cell carcinoma of oropharynx: incidence, localization, and implications for target volume. *Int J Radiat Oncol Biol Phys* 2006; 65: 733 – 738.

[72] Dirix P., Nuyts S., Bussels B., Hermans R., Van den Bogaert W. Prognostic influence of retropharyngeal lymph node metastasis in squamous cell carcinoma of the oropharynx. *Int J Radiat Oncol Biol Phys* 2006; 65: 739 – 744.

In: Dysphagia

Editors: B. S. Smith and M. Adams

ISBN 978-1-61942-104-2

© 2012 Nova Science Publishers, Inc.

Chapter III

Dysphagia in the Myopathies

Danielle Ramos Domenis[1],
Paula de Carvalho Macedo Issa Okubo[1],
Raphaela Barroso Guedes Granzotti[1],
Claudia Ferreira da Rosa Sobreira[2]
and Roberto Oliveira Dantas[3]

[1]Speech Terapist, Departament of Ophtalmology, Otolaryngology and Head and Neck Surgery, University Hospital of Ribeirão Preto, USP, Ribeirão Preto, SP, Brazil
[2]Departament of Neurosciences, Medical School of Ribeirão Preto, USP, Ribeirão Preto, SP, Brazil
[3]Departament of Medicine, Medical School of Ribeirão Preto USP, Ribeirão Preto, SP, Brazil

Abstract

Myopathies are hereditary or acquired diseases of skeletal muscle that result from dysfunction of any constituent of this tissue, leading to the onset of isolated symptoms or combinations of signs and symptoms. There are several types of myopathies, among them inflammatory ones, muscular dystrophies, congenital myopathies, mitochondrial myopathies, and metabolic myopathies. Swallowing is a neurophysiological process whose main function is the efficient transport of food from the mouth to the stomach and which may be divided into four phases: preparatory, oral, pharyngeal, and esophageal. Dysphagia is defined as a set of alterations in any one of these phases, which may cause changes in eating pleasure, malnutrition, dehydration, and even the risk of death. Dysphagia is one of the changes that may be present in myopathies and may vary according to the type of myopathy and the duration of the disease, among other factors. It may appear as an initial symptom or during the course of the disease. Together with cerebrovascular accidents and cranial traumas, neuromuscular diseases are one of the main causes of dysphagia, mainly as a consequence of changes in skeletal muscle directly related to the swallowing process. Speech therapy intervention is essential for dysphagic patients in order to identify factors that increase the risk of tracheal aspiration and to determine ways of avoiding it, thus guaranteeing safe swallowing. This therapy starts with a process of clinical and instrumental evaluation of swallowing. Clinical evaluation is of fundamental importance and guides the indication of objective exams, when necessary, as well as the therapeutic process. Among the objective or complementary methods, videofluoroscopy of swallowing, nasofibrolaryngoscopy and manometry are those most frequently used. After clinical and complementary evaluation it is possible to make an appropriate speech therapy diagnosis and to establish a later conduct regarding the safest feeding route, as well as the indication of rehabilitation or management. Few studies of myopathies have described speech therapy rehabilitation in dysphagia, as well as its efficacy. As is the case for other neurological diseases, it should be kept in mind that the main objective of rehabilitation in the presence of dysphagia often is not the return to, or the maintenance of, feeding by the oral route, but rather the provision of safe nutrition and hydration conditions.

Introduction

The myopathies are hereditary or acquired diseases of skeletal muscle resulting from the dysfunction of any constituent of this tissue, leading to the onset of isolated symptoms or of various combinations of signs and symptoms. Dysphagia can be one of the symptoms present, varying according to time and duration of the disease, in addition to other factors, with the speech therapist being the professional best qualified for its diagnosis and rehabilitation. Knowledge of the disease and of its consequences regarding the biomechanics of swallowing, as well as an appropriate intervention in the patients can prevent eventual cases of dehydration, malnutrition and pulmonary infections.

Anatomophysiology of Swallowing

Swallowing is a physiological process resulting from a complex neuromotor mechanism whose main function is the efficient and safe transport of food from the mouth to the stomach [1]. For this process to occur in an efficient manner, a complex neuromuscular action is necessary, involving sensitivity, taste, proprioception, mobility, and muscular tonus and tension. The integrity of various neuronal systems is essential, such as afferent pathways, integration of stimuli in the central nervous system, efferent pathways, motor response, integrity of the structures involved, and voluntary commands [2].

The central pathway of the spinal cord receives afferences from many central and peripheral pathways which converge to modify the threshold and to evoke the swallowing response. The threshold for evoking swallowing can be intensified by an increased stimulus in the receptor fields of the oropharynx and in the pharyngeal region in particular [3, 4].

The biomechanics of swallowing can be divided into five phases: anticipatory, oral preparatory, oral, pharyngeal, and esophageal [5, 6], which will be described in detail below.

Anticipatory Phase

This phase prepares an individual for the beginning of swallowing and includes a sensory and gustatory stimulus and salivation. Hunger, the visual aspect, olfaction and the environment correspond to the intention and wish to eat, factors that can facilitate or not the next phase, which is the preparatory one [7].

Oral Preparatory Phase

The oral preparatory phase is voluntary and involves manipulation of the bolus inside the mouth and chewing if necessary. Swallowing still starts in the mouth, when the food is voluntarily prepared for swallowing [8]. Physical and chemical characteristics such as volume, consistency, density and degree of humidification are perceived and sent to the central nervous system (CNS), which provides responses related to the propulsive forces of the tongue, of its base and of the pharyngeal body, influencing the pharyngeal phase of swallowing [8, 9, 10, 11].

Mastication is a complex physiological mechanism that involves sequential neuromuscular and digestive sequences and that depends on the pattern of growth, development and maturation of the craniofacial complex, the CNS and the occlusal guides, fundamental aspects for the swallowing and speech function to be performed with efficiency and precision and for the prevention of myofunctional disorders [12]. Mastication can be divided into three phases: incision or bite, trituration and pulverization, and may be unilateral or bilateral, representing a process that permits the appropriate formation of a homogeneous and cohesive food bolus [13].

Oral Phase

This is also a voluntary phase that starts with the coordinated movement of the tongue, favoring the propulsion of the bolus to the pharynx. In addition to elevation and posteriorization of the tongue, there is lip sealing and movement of the soft palate, permitting the food to reach the pharynx. Total sealing of the oral cavity helps the maintenance of the propulsion forces needed to transport the bolus through the hypopharynx and upper esophageal sphincter to the esophagus, a phase that lasts less than one second [14].

Pharyngeal Phase

The pharyngeal phase is involuntary and involves the transport of the food bolus from the oropharynx to the esophagus. Several parameters have been reported in the literature regarding the definition of the pharyngeal phase of swallowing. The pharyngeal phase occurs when the food bolus is pushed to the posterior part of the mouth, stimulating the receptor areas of swallowing, all of them located in the opening of the pharynx, especially in the two tonsillar pillars [15]. Other authors have defined the beginning of the pharyngeal phase as the time when the posterior part of the tongue touches the anterior pillar of the fauces, dislocating the food bolus towards the oropharynx [16]. We may state that the beginning of this phase corresponds to the passage of the food bolus through the posterior region of the nasal spine located at the end of the hard palate, and the end corresponds to the pharyngeal transit of swallowing through the pharyngoesophageal transition [17]. The pharyngeal phase is determined by the pressor transfer from the oral cavity to the pharynx and is elicited by stimuli of receptors at defined sites on the pharyngeal wall [18]. During this phase there is elevation and anteriorization of the larynx, with consequent opening of the pharyngoesophageal transition and passage of the bolus into the esophagus.

Esophageal Phase

The esophageal phase occurs when the esophageal peristalsis formed by the coordinated contraction of striated and smooth muscle carries the bolus to the stomach [19].

Dysphagia in the Myopathies

Dysphagia is any difficulty in swallowing due to an acute or progressive process which may lead to changes in transport of the food bolus from the mouth to the stomach. The condition may be high (oropharyngeal) when there are changes in the oral or pharyngeal phase of swallowing, or low (esophageal) when there are changes in the esophageal phase of swallowing [20]. It is a symptom and not a disease, often representing the first clinical manifestation of an underlying disease [21].

Together with cerebrovascular accidents and head injuries, neuromuscular diseases are among the major causes of dysphagia [22]. This is mainly due to changes in skeletal muscle which are directly related to the swallowing process.

In myopathies, dysphagia may be present due to several factors such as weakness, incoordination, inflammation and other dysfunctions of the oropharyngeal, laryngeal or esophageal muscles [22]. It may appear as the initial symptom or during the course of the disease. The lack of muscle strength may affect one or more phases of swallowing, impairing the process as a whole. There are various types of myopathy, which may have a genetic basis or be acquired. The changes in swallowing that may be present vary widely according to the type of myopathy. Table 1 lists the main types of this condition.

The number of studies regarding the changes in swallowing that occur in the myopathies have increased considerably over the last decades [22, 23, 24]. The main types of myopathy that course with dysphagia are described below.

Table 1. Main types of myopathy

Muscular dystrophies:
Duchenne muscular dystrophy
Becker muscular dystrophy
Limb-girdle muscular dystrophy
Facioscapulohumeral muscular dystrophy
Oculopharyngeal muscular dystrophy
Congenital muscular dystrophies
Myotonic dystrophies
Congenital myopathies
Metabolic myopathies:
Mitochondrial myopathy
Glycogenoses
Disorders of lipid metabolism
Inflammatory myopathies
Endocrine myopathies
Infectious myopathies

Duchenne Muscular Dystrophy (DMD)

This is the most common form of hereditary myopathy in children and also one the most severe, with death likely to occur during the second or third decade of life [25, 26]. It is caused by mutations in the gene encoding the protein dystrophyn, located in the X chromosome, resulting in the absence of the protein. The disease is characterized by progressive muscle weakness resulting in loss of independent ambulation before 13 years of age, with respiratory and cardiac functions being also progressively affected. Over the last few years, the indication of ventilatory support, especially at night, has permitted a longer survival of these patients [27, 28].

Changes in swallowing appear during the more advanced phases of the disease, usually starting from the later years of the second decade of life. Studies have shown that, even though many patients have no complaints about feeding, a specific and objective evaluation shows that they present many changes in the biomechanics of swallowing, to which they are adapted [29]. Dysphagia may be present due to both muscle weakness and to the incoordination between respiration and swallowing, since most patients develop great respiratory difficulties during the course of the disease [30]. The most common alterations present during the more advanced phase of the disease are: changes in mastication mainly as a consequence of the malocclusion present in all patients, altered tongue mobility, weakness of pharyngeal contraction, and residues in the vallecula and piriform recesses. Many patients prefer foods with a softer texture, which is explained mainly by the changes in the preparatory and oral phases of swallowing.

In more serious and advanced cases, when noninvasive ventilation is no longer sufficient, many patients with DMD are submitted to tracheostomy, with the presence of dysphagia being more common. Malnutrition occurs in about 44% of patients, in addition to an increased risk of laryngotracheal aspiration, with the use of gastrostomy as a feeding route being recommended [22, 31, 32].

Myotonic Dystrophy Type 1 (DM1)

DM1, also known as Steinert dystrophy, is a multisystem disease with autosomal dominant pattern of inheritance, caused by a DNA mutation in a protein kinase gene located on the long arm of chromosome 19. It is the most common form of dystrophy among adults. The disease involves the respiratory, cardiac, endocrine, ocular, and central nervous systems in addition to the musculature, which characteristically presents the phenomenon of slower muscle relaxation due to recurrent depolarization of the muscle membrane, called myotonia [33]. The main skeletal muscle related symptoms are progressive muscle weakness ptosis of the eyelids, weakness and atrophy involving the musculature of the face, neck and tongue, and fatigue. The complexity and variability of the disease manifestation make the management of the patient a real challenge regarding management of the patient.

Patients with DM1 present alterations of the stomatognathic system, with facial muscle weakness being perceived on the basis of marked characteristics such as long, triangular and flaccid face [34] present in almost all patients even during the early stages of the disease. The main phonoaudiologic changes that may be present in DM1 are dysphonia, dysarthria and dysphagia, resulting from the atrophy, weakness and fatigability of the oropharyngeal and laryngeal muscles [35, 36, 37].

Dysphagia should be well investigated since it may be one of the factors responsible for the occurrence of pneumonia, this being one of the main causes of death during advanced stages of the disease [35, 38]. The difficulties are mainly present in the preparatory and oral phases and consist of masticatory inefficiency and inadequate formation of the food bolus and its ejection. Weakness of pharyngeal contraction is also observed. These changes compromise the entire biomechanics of swallowing, increasing the risk of laryngotracheal aspiration.

Oculopharyngeal Muscular Dystrophy (OPMD)

OPMD is a hereditary disease with manifestations of late onset, usually around the 4th and 6th decade of life, of slow progression and having ptosis of the eyelids and dysphagia as the main characteristics. In more advanced stages, extraocular and facial muscles may also be affected [39].

The early symptoms of the disease may be phonoaudiologic, being often perceived before a full diagnosis is made, consisting of aphony or voice changes, articulatory changes and dysphagia. Aspiration pneumonia is one of the main causes of death during the advanced stages of the disease. Studies have shown that the main signs of many patients are oral and nasal reflux, coughing and choking while eating, weight loss, recurrent pulmonary infections, and a sensation of food stuck in the throat. Many patients present changes in the cricopharyngeal region that cause reflux and aspiration of the refluxed content [40]. Other studies using esophageal manometry have shown that most patients with OPMD have a reduction of esophageal peristalsis, often presenting changes in both smooth and striated muscle. Other characteristics of these patients are weakness of pharyngeal contractions, simultaneous contractions and incomplete relaxation of the esophagus determined by manometry [41, 42, 43]. The use of compensatory maneuvers and changes in the diet improve the quality of life of these patients and reduce the risks of aspiration. Surgical procedures trying to improve the functioning of the region of the pharyngoesophageal transition have not been very successful [44].

Inflammatory Myopathy

This is a group of acquired muscle diseases characterized by muscle weakness of subacute or chronic onset due to inflammation in skeletal muscle. The idiopathic inflammatory myopathies consists of polymyositis (PM), dermatomyositis (DM) and inclusion body myositis (IBM). Each one of the three diseases has specific characteristics as well as pathogenesis and patterns of muscle weakness [45, 46]. DM differs from PM also by presenting skin inflammation. In IBM, disease progression is slower, with an asymmetric pattern and a greater predominance in men. Dysphagia is one of the main characteristics of the disease [47, 48, 49].

Dysphagia is a frequent symptom, occurring in up to 60% of the patients during the subacute phase of inflammatory myopathies. The main complaints of the patients are: a sensation of dry mouth, food stuck in the throat, coughing and choking when eating, and difficulty with solid and dry foods. The main changes detected in several studies were weakness and incoordination of the tongue, important reduction of laryngeal elevation and of the whole hyolaryngeal complex, reduction of the cricopharyngeal opening, involvement of the skeletal and smooth muscle of the esophagus causing dysmotility and delayed esophageal emptying, reflux with frequent aspiration of the refluxed content, and nasal regurgitation [49, 50, 51]. In these patients the prognosis of dysphagia is poor during the subacute phase, with drug treatment of the disease having little effect on these symptoms [22, 52]. The best therapeutic intervention is adequacy of feeding, swallowing exercises including the Mendelsohn maneuver, in addition to myotomy of the cricopharyngeal muscle and pharyngoesophageal dilatation [53, 54]. Aspiration pneumonia is a cause of death, as also observed in other myopathies [49].

Mitochondrial Myopathy (MM)

MM represents a group of clinically heterogeneous disorders that may affect multiple systems in addition to skeletal muscle. They may cause muscle involvement with clinical characteristics of delayed motor acquisition, developmental regression, hypotonia, proximal weakness, ptosis, and progressive external ophthalmoplegia. Fatigability may be the main complaint, being clearly disproportional to the degree of muscle weakness and atrophy detected. There is no pattern of muscle weakness and atrophy in the limbs, with proximal, distal or diffuse involvement being detected. Muscle weakness may be responsible for respiratory insufficiency. The signs and symptoms may be stationary, progressive or episodic in both sexes, in any age range, and may be sporadic or familial. Muscle involvement may be the mode of presentation of the disease, may be an isolated symptom or be accompanied by involvement of other organs and systems such as the nervous and endocrine systems, the liver, heart, retina and kidney [55, 56]. Among the manifestations related to skeletal muscle there is development of progressive external ophthalmoplegia, proximal or generalized muscle weakness, myalgia, and early fatigue. Other common signs are short stature, sensorineural deafness, optic atrophy, ataxia, epilepsy, peripheral neuropathy, and progressive encephalopathy, among others.

Symptoms of dysphagia in MM have been cited by many authors [57, 58, 59, 60], but investigations for the characterization of swallowing changes are scarce. The main complaints concern solid and dry foods and involve a sensation of food stuck in the throat, the need to swallow several times, and the use of liquids to help with dry foods. The main changes detected are: nasal reflux, prolonged oral preparatory phase, reduced tongue propulsion, and residues in the vallecula and piriform recesses mainly involving solid foods [61, 62, 63].

Phonoaudiologic Evaluation of Dysphagia

Care for the dysphagic patient starts with the process of evaluation which consists of directed anamnesis followed by clinical evaluation for the analysis of the structures that participate in the dynamics of swallowing. To this end, the examiner must have knowledge about the anatomical structures and the neurophysiological processes involved in swallowing, which is important for the understanding of the relation between phases and for the determination of the clinical therapeutic reasoning [64].

Anamnesis

Anamnesis aims to understand the diagnosis of the disease and its clinical antecedents. In progressive diseases such as myopathies, it is very important to obtain information about the time of disease onset and its time course. Nutritional, pulmonary and cognitive aspects, as well as he medications used should be recorded.

Regarding swallowing and other phonoaudiologic aspects, the complaints reported by the patient and by his relatives or persons living with him must be investigated. In addition to recording the complaints reported by the patient, it is important to apply a directed questionnaire containing specific questions related to swallowing. Studies have shown that many patients, by having been sick for a long time, learn to live with some symptoms without perceiving them as alterations, spontaneously modifying the consistency of their food and even performing compensatory maneuvers. A specific questionnaire is of help for a better understanding of the possible changes in the dynamics of swallowing, and could be used as a tool predictive of dysphagia, when present [65, 66].

Clinical Phonoaudiologic Evaluation

During clinical evaluation, the facial structures and all structures involved in the biomechanics of swallowing should be first observed, characterizing the aspect of the face, the presence or absence of atrophies, the status of tooth conservation and occlusion, and the mobility and tonus of facial muscles, of mastication, soft palate and tongue.

In addition to structural evaluation, when possible, functional evaluation is performed using food. Priority is given to the foods that are part of the daily life of the patient, as well as to utensils and maneuvers already used by him. During swallowing, the examiner observes lip sealing, oral containment, mastication, presence of nasal reflux, laryngeal elevation, presence of residues, presence of multiple swallows, coughing, choking or throat clearing, and changes in respiration. Some tools that can help clinical evaluation are available, contributing to the reasoning related to the prediction of whether the patient is aspirating the food evaluated. They are the stethoscope, which permits cervical auscultation, and the pulse oximeter. After evaluation, the speech therapist should be able to conclude whether or not the patient can safely eat by the oral route. There are many classifications of the signs and symptoms of dysphagia and of its severity. However, more than classifying, a professional should be able to apply a clinical reasoning to what is happening and to determine how he can help his patient regarding the maintenance of nutrition and hydration status, as well as regarding protection against pulmonary infections [2, 67, 68, 69, 70, 71, 72, 73].

There has been much discussion about the efficiency of clinical evaluation as the main instrument for the diagnosis of dysphagias, and it has been increasingly observed that, despite its limitations, clinical evaluation guides the indication of objective exams and helps the therapeutic process [67, 74, 75, 76].

Complementary Exams

Clinical evaluation is not always sufficient to define the presence or absence of aspiration, especially when aspiration is silent [74]. Thus, some complementary exams can be used, with nasofibrolaryngoscopy and videofluoroscopy of swallowing being the two most frequently employed. Other complementary exams are esophageal manometry, scintigraphy and surface electromyography. Esophageal manometry is used for the study of esophageal functioning and not directly for the detection of laryngotracheal aspiration. Scintigraphy is a simple, noninvasive and safe technique that can quantitate the passage of the bolus through the oropharynx and that can provide a measurement of the bolus in a given region. However, its diagnostic accuracy is low since the procedure does not permit a detailed visualization of the structures during the swallowing process, being mainly used in research. Surface electromyography can be used for diagnosis and also as a therapeutic instrument, quantitating the functioning of determined muscle structures involved in swallowing.

The objective of nasofibrolaryngoscopy is to observe the characteristics of the mucosa, to evaluate the anatomical structures of the pharynx and larynx in terms of mobility and sensitivity, as well as the functionality of swallowing. Although invasive, it is a simple and safe method which can also be used by the bedside. The objective of the exam is to locate topographically the most evident and significant changes occurring during the swallowing function [77].

The videofluoroscopy of swallowing is considered to be the gold standard exam for the study of oropharyngeal dysphagia since, in addition to detecting the presence of aspiration or microaspiration, it permits the dynamic observation of the structures involved in swallowing during the various phases of the process [67, 78, 79, 80, 81]. The videofluoroscopy of swallowing has various advantages such as the possibility of a precise and immediate analysis of swallowing in various positions, low cost, a noninvasive procedure whose results can be analyzed later, and the possibility of an objective measurement with a computer program. Among the disadvantages are: exposure to radiation, use of barium and the impossibility to visualize structural anomalies such as hyperemia and tumors [82]. The exam is contraindicated in cases in which laryngotracheal aspiration is evident and when the exam does not permit a direct assessment of the sensitivity of the pharyngolaryngeal region.

Phonoaudiologic Rehabilitation

After a diagnostic definition based on clinical and complementary evaluation, the primary step is for the multidisciplinary team to determine the safest feeding route for the patient.

In the case of the indication of feeding by an alternative route for patients with a diagnosis of myopathy, gastrostomy should be considered by the team, since these diseases are progressive and tend to worsen with time and the rehabilitation process may be long. The primordial objective of rehabilitation in dysphagia is to enable efficient swallowing in order to reintroduce oral feeding without posing risks to the patient. It consists of the selection of a group of appropriate therapeutic techniques and strategies for the patient in question, mainly aiming at his general well-being, with the maintenance of adequate pulmonary, nutritional and hydration conditions without overlooking the rescue of eating pleasure [67]. Therapy for dysphagic patients may be indirect when it involves techniques with no food offered in order to improve the mobility and sensitivity of structures related to the dynamics of swallowing, and direct when food is offered.

Among the procedures used for rehabilitation are: changes of the utensils used for eating, adequate preparation of the environment and of food consistency, use of postural and compensatory maneuvers, guidelines about oral hygiene, and execution of specific techniques and exercises according to the changes presented by the patient. In view of the variety of symptoms and the differences between myopathy types, it was not the objective of the present chapter to teach specific techniques for the rehabilitation of swallowing in myopathies. There is no prescription or rigid rule to be followed in a generalized manner, but knowledge about the diagnosis and prognosis and especially the expectations of the patient and his relatives is very important. Before starting rehabilitation, it is important for the entire family to be involved and to be aware of the full therapeutic process and of the fundamental role of the family for the result of the intervention. Research involving rehabilitation and its efficacy in the dysphagias is recent and almost nonexistent in neuromuscular diseases, myopathies in particular. It is the task of the speech therapist and of the entire team of professionals who deal with these still incurable or untreatable diseases to find the courage to continue to look for responses that may provide a better quality of life for the patients.

References

[1]   Macedo-Filho, ED. Conceitos e fisiologia aplicada da deglutição. In: Macedo-Filho, Ed; Pisani, JC; Carneiro, JE; Gomes, G. *Disfagia: abordagem multidisciplinar*. 3ª ed. Rio de Janeiro: Frontis, 1999; p 3-8.

[2]   Furkim, AM; Silva, RG. *Programas de reabilitação em disfagia neurogênica*. São Paulo: Frôntis Editorial; 1999.

[3]   Miller, AJ. Deglutition. *Physiol Rev*. 1982; 62: 129-184.

[4]   Miller, AJ. Neurophysiological basis of swallowing. *Dysphagia*. 1986; 1: 91-100.

[5]   Leopold, NA, Kagel, MC. Dysphagia – ingestion or deglutition?: a proposed paradigm. *Dysphagia*. 1997; 12: 202-6.

[6]   Haber, SN. The primate basal ganglia: parallel and integrative networks. *J. Chem. Neuroanat*. 2003; 26: 317-30.

[7]   Ferreira, LP; Befi-Lopes, BM; Limongi, SCO. Tratado de Fonoaudiologia. Edit Roca, 2004.

[8]   Costa, MMB. Dinâmica da deglutição: fase oral e faríngea. In: COSTA, MMB; Leme, E; Kock, HI. *Colóquio multidisciplinar deglutição and disfagia*. Rio de Janeiro, 1998.

[9]   Dantas, RO; Dodds, WJ; Massey, BT; Kern, MK. The effect of high-vs low density barium preparations on the quantitative features of swallowing. *AJR Am. J. Roentgenol* 1989; 153: 1191-1195.

[10] Dantas, RO; Dodds, WJ. Influência da viscosidade do bolo alimentar deglutido na motilidade da faringe. Arq. *Gastroenterol* 1990; 127: 164-168.

[11] Logemann JA; Kahrilas PJ; Cheng J; Pauloski BR; Gibbons PJ; Rademaker AW; LIN S. Closure mechanisms of the laryngeal vestibule during swallowing. *Am. J. Physiol* 1992; 262: G338-G344.

[12] Tanigute, CC. Desenvolvimento das funções estomatognáticas. In: Marchesan, IQ. *Fundamentos em fonoaudiologia: aspectos clínicos da motricidade oral*. Rio de Janeiro: Guanabara Koogan; 1998. 1-6.

[13] Bianchini EMG. Mastigação e ATM: avaliação e terapia. In: Marchesan, IQ. *Fundamentos em fonoaudiologia: aspectos clínicos da motricidade oral*. Rio de Janeiro Koogan; 1998. 37-49.

[14] Marchesan, IQ. Deglutição: normalidade. In: Furkim, AM; Santini, CS. *Disfagias Orofaríngeas*. Carapicuíba: Pró-Fono, 1999. 3-18.

[15] Giyton, AC. *Tratado de Fisiologia Médica*. 7ª ed. Philadelphia: Guanabara-Koogan; 1986. 603-604.

[16] Dodds, WJ; Stewart, ED; Logemann, JA. Physiology and radiology of the normal oral and pharyngeal phases of swallowing. *AJR*. 1990; 154: 953-963.

[17] Kendall, KA; Mckenzie, S; Leonard, RJ; Gonçalves, MI; Walker, A. Timing of events in normal swallowing: a videofluoroscopic study. *Dysphagia*. 2000; 15: 74-83.

[18] Costa, MMB. Avaliação da dinâmica da deglutição e da disfagia orofaríngea. In: Castro, LP; Savassi-Rocha, PR; MELO, JRC; COSTA, MMB. *Tópicos em Gastroenterologia*. Rio de Janeiro: Médica e Científica Ltda; 2000; 177-185.

[19] Logemann, JA. *Evaluation and treatment of swallowing disorders*. Austin: Pro- ed; 1983.

[20] Macedo-Filho, ED; Gomes GF; Furkim AM. *Manual de cuidados do paciente com disfagia*. São Paulo: Lovise; 2000.

[21] Marchesan, IQ. Disfagia. In: Marchesan, IQ; Bolaffi, G; Gomes, ICD; Zorzi, JL. *Tópicos em Fonoaudiologia 1995*. São Paulo: Lovise, 1995: 161-166.

[22] Sonies, BC. Evaluation and treatment of speech and swallowing disorders associated with myopathies. *Current Opinion in Rheumatology*. 1997, 9: 486-495.

[23] Willig, TN; Paulus, J; Saint-Guily, JL; Béon, C; Navarro, J. Swallowing problems in neuromuscular disorders. *Arch. Phys. Med. Rehabil.* 1994; 75: 1175- 1181.

[24] Leonard, RJ; Kendall, KA; Johnson, R; Mckenzie, S. Swallowing in myotonic muscular dystrophy: A videofluoroscopic study. *Arch. Phys. Med. Rehabil*, 2001, july 82; 979-985.

[25] Emery, AEH. Population frequencies of inherited neuromuscular disease – a world survey. *Neuromusc Disord*, 1991; 1: 19-29.

[26] Dubowitz, V. Muscle disorders in childhood. 2nd ed, 1995.

[27] Eagle, M; Baudouin, SV; Chandler, C; Giddings, DR; Bullock, R; Bushby, K. Survival in Duchenne muscular dystrophy: improvements in life expectancy since 1967 and the impact of home nocturnal ventilation. *Neuromuscul Disord*, 2002; 12: 926-929.

[28] Kohler, M; Clarenbach, CF; Bahler, C; Brack, T; Russi, EW; Bloch, KE. Disability and survival in Duchenne muscular dystrophy. *J. Neurol. Neurosurg. Psychiatry*, 2009; 80; 320-325.

[29] Shinonaga, C; Fukuda, M; Suzieki, Y; Higaki, T; Ishida, Y; Ishii, E; Hyodo, M; Morimoto, T; Sano, N. Letter to the Editor- Evaluation of swallowing function in Duchenne muscular dystrophy. *Developmental Medicine and Child Neurology*, 2008; 50: 478-480.

[30] Pane, M; Vasta, I; Messina, S; Sorleti, D; Aloysius, A; Sciarra, F; Mangiola, F; Kinali, M; Ricci, E; Mercuri, E. Feeding problems and weight gain in Duchenne muscular dystrophy. *Eur. J. Paediatr. Neurol*, 2006; 10: 231-236.

[31] Willig, TN; Bach, JR; Venance, V; Navarro, J. Nutritional rehabilitation in neuromuscular disorders. *Semin. Neurol.* 1995; 15: 18-23.

[32] Terzi, N; Prigent, H; Lejaille, M; Falaize, L; Annane, D; Orlikowski, D; Lofaso, F. Impact of tracheostomy on swallowing performance in Duchenne muscular dystrophy. *Neuromuscul Disord*, 2010; Aug 20(8): 493-498.

[33] Harper, P. Myotonic dystrophy. 3rd ed. London: WB Saunders; 2001.

[34] Staley, RN; Bishara, SE; Hanson, JW; Nowak, AJ. Craniofacial development in myotonic dystrophy. *Cleft Palate Craniofac. J* 1992; 29: 456-462.

[35] Chiappeta, ALML; Oda, AL; Zanoteli, E; Guilherme, A; OLIVEiRA, ASB. Disfagia orofaríngea na distrofia miotônica: avaliação fonoaudiológica e análise nasofibrolaringoscópica. *Arqu neuropsiquiatr.* 2001; 59: 394-400.

[36] Noronha, CFC; Duro, LAA. Avaliação orofacial através de uma escala de pontuação em pacientes com distrofia miotônica (doença de Steinert). *Arq. Neuropsiquiatr.* 1995; 53: 424-431.

[37] Lichtenfels-Rodrigues, E; Buiatti, VP; Chiappetta, ALML; Oliveira, AB. A efetividade das orientações fonoaudiológicas em pacientes com distrofia miotônica tipo 1 (DM1). *Rev. Cefac.* 2003; 5: 329-334.

[38] Mathieu, J; Allard, P; Potvin, L; Prevost, C; Begin, P. A 10-year study of mortality in a cohort of patients with myotonic dystrophy. *Neurology* 1999; 52: 1658-1662.

[39] Munitiz, V; Ortiz, A; Martinez De Haro, LF. Diagnosis and treatment of oculopharyngeal dystrophy: a report of three cases from the same family. *Dis. Esophagus.* 2003; 16: 160-164.

[40] Lim, CT; Chew, CT; Chew, SH. Oculopharyngeal muscular dystrophy: a case report and a review of literature. *Ann. Acad. Med* 1992; 21:399-403.

[41] Tiomny, E; Khikevic, O; Korozyn, AD; Kimmel, R; Hallack, A; Baron, J; Blumen, S; Asherov, A; Gilat, T. Esophageal smooth muscle dysfunction in oculopharyngeal muscular dystrophy. *Dig. Dis. Sci.* 1996; 41: 1350-1354.

[42] Duranceau, CA; Letendre, J; Clermont, RJ; Levesque, H; Barbeau, A. Oropharyngeal dysphagia in patients with oculopharyngeal muscular dystrophy. *Can. J. Surg.* 1978; 21(4) 326-329.

[43] Castell, JA; Castell, DO; Duranceau, CA; Topart, P. Manometric characteristics of the pharynx, upper esophageal sphincter, esophagus, and lower esophageal sphincter in patients with oculopharyngeal muscular dystrophy. *Dysphagia* 1995; 10:22-26.

[44] Buchholz, DW. Cricopharyngeal myotomy may be effective treatment for selected patients with neurogenic oropharyngeal dysphagia. *Dysphagia* 1995; 10:255-258.

[45] Dalakas, MC. Polymyositis, dermatomyositis and inclusion- bady myositis. *N. Engl. J. Méd* 1991; 325: 1487.

[46] Mastaglia, FL. Inflammatory muscle diseases. *Neurol India.* 2008; 56(3): 263-270.

[47] Ringel, S; Kenny, C; Neville, H; Giorno, R; Carry, M. Spectrum of inclusion body myositis. *Arch Neurol.* 1987, 44: 1154-1157.

[48] Lotz, BP; Engel, AG; Nishino, H; Stevens, JC; Litchy, WJ. Inclusion body myositis. *Brain* 1989, 112: 727-747.

[49] Oh, TH; Brumfield, KA; Hoskin, TL; Stolp, KA; Murray, JA; Bassford, JR. Dysphagia in inflammatory myopathy: clinical characteristics, treatment strategies, and outcome in 62 patients. *Mayo. Clin. Proc.* 2007; 82: 441-447.

[50] Williams, RB; Grehan, MJ; Hersch, M; Andre, J; Cook, IJ. Biomechanics, diagnosis, and treatment outcome in inflammatory myopathy presenting as oropharyngeal dysphagia. *Gut* 2003; 52: 471-478.

[51] Kim, SJ; Han, TR; Jeong, SJ; Beom, JW. Comparison between swallowing-related and limb muscle involvement in dermatomyositis patients. *Scand. J. Rheumatol.* 2010; 39: 336-340.

[52] Kagen, LJ; Hochman, RB; Strong, EW. Cricopharyngeal obstruction in inflammatory myopathy (polymyositis/dermatomyositis). *Arthritis Rheum.* 1985, 28: 630-636.

[53] Miller, RM; Langmore, SE. Treatment efficacy for adults with oropharyngeal dysphagia. *Arch. Phys. Med. Rehabil.* 1994; 75: 1256-1262.

[54] Langmore, SE; Miller, RM. Behavioral treatment for adults with oropharyngeal dysphagia. *Arch. Phys. Med. Rehabil.* 1994; 75: 1154-1160.

[55] Dimauro, S; Bonilla, E; Zeviani, M; Nakagawa, M; De Vivo, DC. Mitochondrial myopathies. Ann Neurol. 1985; 17: 521-538.

[56] Dias-Tosta, E. Citopatias mitocondriais: aspectos clínicos. *Rev. Bras. Neurol.* 1994; 30(1): 3-8.

[57] Vu, TH; Sciacco, M; Tanji, K; Nichter, C; Bonilla, E; Chatkupt, S; Maertens, P; Shanske, S; Mendell, J; Koenigsberger, MR; Sharer, L; Schon, EA; Dimauro, S; Devivo, DC. Clinical manifestations of mitochondrial DNA depletion. *Neurology.* 1998; 50: 1783-1790.

[58] Garcidueñas, ALC; Loria, OP; Sagastegui, JA; Garcia, RF. Oftalmoplegia progressiva externa secundaria a miopatia mitocondrial. Presentación de um caso y revisión de la literatura. *Gac. Med. Mex.* 2000; 136(3): 267-271.

[59] Klopstock, T; Jaksch, M; Gasser, T. Age and cause of death in mitochondrial diseases. *Neurology.* 1999, 53(4): 855-857.

[60] Jimenez-Caballero, PE; Serviá, M; Cabeza, CI; Marsal-Alonso, C; Alvarez-Tejerina, A. Chronic progressive external ophthalmoplegia: clinical and electromyographic manifestations in a series of cases. *Rev. Neurol.,* 2006, dec- 16-31; 43(12): 724-728.

[61] Kornblum, C; Broicher, R; Walther, E; Seibel, P; Reichmann, H; Klockgether, T; Herberhold, C; Schroder, R. Cricopharyngeal achalasia is a common cause of dysphagia in patients with mtDNA deletions. *Neurology.* 2001, 56(10): 1409-1412.

[62] Katsanos, KH; Nastos, D; Noussias, V; Christodoulou, D; Kappas, A; Tsianos, EV. Manometric study in Kearns-Sayre syndrome. *Dis. of the Esophagus,* 2001, 14(1), p.63-66.

[63] Domenis DR. Estudo da deglutição em pacientes com miopatia mitocondrial do tipo oftalmoplegia externa crônica progressiva: avaliação clínica, manométrica e videofluoroscópica. Dissertação de Mestrado – Faculdade de Medicina da Universidade de São Paulo; 2008.

[64] Silva, RG; Gatto, AR; Cola, PC. Disfagia Orofaríngea neurogênica em adultos- avaliação fonoaudiológica em leito hospitalar. In: JACOBI, JS; Levy, DS; Silva, LMC. Disfagia Avaliação e Tratamento. Rio de Janeiro. *Revinter,* 2003; 181-196.

[65] Cox, FM; Verschuuren, JJ; Verbist, BM; Niks, EH; Wintzen, AR; Badrising, UA. Detecting dysphagia in inclusion body myositis. *J. Neurol.* 2009; 256: 2009-2013.

[66] Mulcahy, KP; Langdon, PC; Mastaglia, F. Dysphagia in inflammatory myopathy: self-report, incidence, and prevalence. *Dysphagia,* 2011 (online).

[67] Chiappetta, ALML; ODA, AL. Disfagia Orofaríngea Neurogênica. In: Levy, JA; Oliveira, ASB. Reabilitação em Doenças Neurológicas - Guia Terapêutico Prático. São Paulo: *Editora Atheneu,* 2003; 81-92.

[68] Santoro, P; Silva, IL; Cardoso, F; Dias JUNIOR, E; Beresford, H. Evaluation of the effectiveness of a phonoaudiology program for the rehabilitation of dysphagia in the elderly. *Archives of Gerontology and Geriatrics,* 2011; 53(1): 61-66.

[69] Daniels, SK; McAdam, CP; Brailey, K; Foundas, AL. Clinical assessment of swallowing and prediction of dysphagia severity. *Am. J. Speech Lang Pathol.* 1997; 6(4): 17-22.

[70] Salassa, JR. A functional outcome swallowing scale for staging oropharyngeal dysphagia. *Dig Dis.* 1999; 17(4): 230-234.

[71] O'Neil, KH; Purdy, M; Falk, J; Gallo, L. The dysphagia outcome and severity scale. *Dysphagia.* 1999; 14(3): 139-145.

[72] Padovani, AR; Moraes, DP; Mangili, LD; Andrade, CRF. Protocolo fonoaudiológico de avaliação do risco para disfagia (PARD). *Rev. Soc. Bras. Fonoaudiol.* 2007; 12(3): 199-205.

[73] Crary, MA; Mann, GD; Groher, ME. Initial psychometric assessment of a functional oral intake scale for dysphagia in stroke patients. *Arch. Phys. Med. Rehabil.* 2005; 86(8): 1516-1520.

[74] Linden, P; Siebens, AA. Dysphagia: predicting laryngeal penetration. *Arch. Phys. Med,* 1983: 64; 282-284.

[75] Mathers- Schmidt, BA; KURLiNSKI, M. Dysphagia evaluation practices: inconsistencies in clinical assessment and instrumental examination decision-making. *Dysphagia,* 2003. Spring; 18 (2): 114-125.

[76] Miller, RM. Clinical examination for dysphagia. In: GROHER, ME. *Dysphagia: Diagnosis and Management.* 2nd ed. Boston, 1992; 143-162.

[77] Barros, AFF; Okubo, PCMI; Domenis, DR; Ricz, HM; Mello-Filho, FV. Comparação entre a avaliação clínica e objetiva da deglutição em pacientes com disfagia orofaríngea neurogênica. *Rev. Soc. Brás. Fonoaudiol.* 2006, 11(2): 90-95.

[78] Manrique, D. Avaliação otorrinolaringológica da deglutição. In: Furkim, AM; Santini, CS. Disfagias Orofaríngeas. Carapicuíba, SP. *Pró Fono,* 1999; 49-60.

[79] Beck, JT; Gayler, BW. Image quality and radiation levels in videofluoroscopy for swallowing studies: a Review. *Dysphagia.* 1990; (5): 118-128.

[80] Costa, MMB; Nova, JLL; Carlos, MT; Pereira, AP; Koch, HA. Videofluoroscopia – um novo método. *Radiol Bras* 1992; 25: 11-18.

[81] Costa, M; Monteiro, JS. Exame videofluoroscópico das fases oral e faríngea da deglutição. In: Costa, M; Castro, LP. Tópicos em deglutição e disfagia. Rio de Janeiro: *MEDSI* 2003; 273-284.

[82] Gonçalves, MIR; Vidigal, MLN. Avaliação videofluoroscópica das disfagias. In: Disfagias Orofaríngeas. Carapicuíba, SP: *Pró-Fono,* 1999: 189-202.

In: Dysphagia ISBN 978-1-61942-104-2
Editors: B. S. Smith and M. Adams © 2012 Nova Science Publishers, Inc.

Chapter IV

Swallow Screening as an Essential Component of Acute Stroke Management

Julie Luker and Kylie Wall
International Centre for Allied Health Evidence, University of South
Australia, Adelaide, South Australia

Abstract

Dysphagia following stroke is common and increases patient risk of
poor outcomes and adverse events. Swallow screening is an important
process of care for patients who suffer acute stroke. This brief
examination aims to identify those patients that may be at risk of
swallowing problems so that comprehensive assessment and management
can be provided. However, despite wide agreement that swallow
screening is an essential component of care, there is no agreement
regarding how or when screening should be performed, and by whom.
Debate continues regarding the validity and reliability of various
screening tools, and whether they are able to provide an acceptable level
of certainty in risk detection. Our chapter reviews the current evidence
underpinning swallow screening for acute stroke patients.

Published clinical quality audits on acute stroke populations have
reported suboptimal compliance with swallow screening. Current
evidence suggests that multiple factors contribute to screening
compliance, including the structures and systems within health care

facilities, such as stroke unit care. The provision of swallow screening may also be influenced by demographic and stroke-related variables of the patients themselves, such age, gender and stroke severity.

The results of the authors' recent research on the factors that influence the quality of stroke swallow screening will be presented. This was conducted in three Australian tertiary hospitals. The study retrospectively audited the care provided to 300 patients admitted with acute stroke. Data was collected on swallow screen compliance and other variables of interest including stroke unit admission, day of admission, patients' age, gender, English proficiency, comorbidities, pre-stroke levels of independence and type of accommodation, stroke severity and length of stay. Logistical univariate and multivariate stepwise regression analysis was undertaken to explore the determinants of screening compliance in this population. In the sample, patients with milder stroke, and those admitted over a weekend, were at increased risk of not receiving a swallow screen.

Swallow screening is an accepted care process in acute stroke management, despite ongoing debate regarding the best way to conduct the screening. Studies, including our own, report suboptimal provision of swallow screening. The factors that influence swallow screening compliance may be complex and include variables within hospital systems, as well as variables related to the patient and their stroke.

Introduction

Stroke is a major health issue internationally. In Australia alone around 60,000 people suffer stroke annually making it the country's second greatest cause of death and the leading cause of disability [1, 2]. The past decade has seen an increase in research evidence regarding the best care for acute stroke patients, aimed at optimising their outcomes. This has led to the development of high quality stroke guidelines to steer clinical care [3]. Guideline recommendations encompass the prevention of complications associated with stroke-related mortality and other poor outcomes [4].

Oropharyngeal dysphagia is a common consequence of stroke and it increases patient risk of post-stroke complications. Reported incidence of dysphagia varies, with an Australian national audit reporting 47% [5], and instrumental videofluoroscopic examination reporting that dysphagia affects 64 − 78% of stroke patients [6]. About half of these patients with dysphagia will recover a functional swallow within a week, but the remainder may experience dysphagia for several months or longer [6, 7]. A systematic review and meta-analysis conducted by Martino's group [6] confirmed that patients presenting with dysphagia had a significantly increased risk of developing pneumonia (RR 3.17; 95% CI 3.3-39.7]. Dysphagia is also associated with increased risk of malnutrition and dehydration, increased length of stay and in-hospital death [6, 8, 9]. Given the serious potential consequences of dysphagia, it is unsurprising that the detection, assessment and management of this condition is prominent in stroke guidelines.

The provision of routine swallow screening had been shown to improve patient outcomes and reduce the occurrence of pneumonia following acute stroke [10, 11]. However, despite wide agreement that swallow screening is an essential component of care, there is no agreement regarding how or when screening should be performed, and by whom.

In this chapter, swallow screening is defined as a brief examination of swallow function which aims to detect patients who may be at risk of swallowing problems so that comprehensive assessment and management can be provided. Patients found to have a safe swallow at screening can commence oral intake without the delay of waiting for a specialist assessment [12]. Screening is often administered by non-specialists in dysphagia including nursing staff, or any other member of the multi-disciplinary team. Ideally, screening requires minimal training to educate the screening staff on the basic understanding of dysphagia and administration of the screening tool.

In this chapter screening is differentiated from a comprehensive bedside swallow assessment, which is defined as a more detailed procedure performed by clinicians with specialised knowledge in dysphagia and skills in interpreting findings, such as a speech pathologist.

When to Screen and by whom?

We recently conducted a systematic review on the use of process indicators to determine the quality of care provided to patients with dysphagia following acute stroke [13]. All 21 reviewed articles used process indicators for swallow screening as a measure of quality stroke care. However there was no agreement regarding the optimal timing of screening: seven articles specified screening performed before oral intake, seven used a timeframe of within 24 hours of admission, while seven authors did not mention timing as a quality-of-care consideration. As most of the reviewed articles were retrospective studies, it is possible that this equivocal evidence on the best time to screen reflected pragmatic difficulties of collecting retrospective data on oral intake, rather than sound evidence of effectiveness. *A priory* reasoning would suggest that oral intake should be forestalled until a safe swallow is confirmed, and this is in fact reflected in recent clinical guideline recommendations [3](p82).

There are no current evidence-based recommendations for the level of training required to perform a swallow screen. Australia's Clinical Guidelines for Stroke Management simply specify that "Personnel specifically trained in swallow screening using a validated tool should undertake screening" [3](p82). Speech Pathologists or Speech & Language Therapists (SPs) are recognised experts in the assessment and management of dysphagia [14]. However, given the requirement for rapid swallow screening for all stroke admissions over seven days a week, allocating this role to SPs is an inefficient use of resources [12]. Emerging evidence suggests that training nursing staff to conduct swallow screening is a feasible option. Cichero's study [12] with stroke and non-stroke patients reported that nurses who undertook a detailed training program conducted by SPs were able to adequately detect the risk of dyspahagia on screening. Compared to repeated screening conducted by SPs, nurse-screening had 95% sensitivity and 97% specificity. This is supported by the Weinhardt et al [15] study, where 94% agreement was demonstrated in swallow screen results when conducted by registered nurses and SP staff with a population of acute stroke patients.

Screening Tools Available

Debate continues regarding the validity and reliability of various screening tools and whether they are able to provide an acceptable level of certainty in dysphagia detection. Current stroke clinical guidelines have been unable to make many specific recommendations due to a lack of clarity in the underpinning evidence [3, 6]. A large number of studies have attempted to establish the most valuable screening tools, however flawed methodological quality and variability between studies has failed to lead to a unanimous conclusion [6, 10].

The accuracy of swallow screening in detecting stroke related dysphagia is particularly difficult for the proportion of patients who exhibit no overt signs of aspiration, such as coughing. This silent aspiration has been reported in 28-52% of acute stroke patients [16]. The Nakajoh et al (2000) study on stroke patients revealed that the latency of the cough reflex was significantly associated with the incidence of pneumonia [17]. Therefore screening tools that depend on an overt cough response to penetration and/or aspiration may miss many stroke patients who are at risk.

Variable information is available on the psychometric properties of some swallow screening tools. Determining validity, sensitivity and specificity relies on the ability to compare findings from screening tools to a recognised 'gold standard' however agreement on a reference standard for detecting post-stroke aspiration has been problematic [18]. While videofluroscopy (VFS) has been long considered the reference standard for swallow assessment [19], this is not unanimously accepted for acute stroke patients [18]. Problems exist with the feasibility of using VFS following stroke, especially for severely affected patients with poor sitting balance. Furthermor the inter-rater reliability data on VFS to detect dysphagia is also poor [20, 21], and evidence is still emerging regarding the best materials and measurement tools to use during testing [22, 23]. Fiberoptic endoscopic evaluation of swallow (FEES) is an alternative reference standard for swallowing screening, and FEES has demonstrated sensitivity and specificity values which are comparable to VFS. Although it is an invasive procedure, FEES may be more feasible for use in acute stroke due to bedside portability and reduced radiation exposure [24]. Whether using FEES or VFS as the reference test, recent validation studies use penetration to the level of vocal folds and/or aspiration as the end point of testing [25].

Intermittent systematic reviews have tracked the availability of new swallow screening tools over time [18, 25-27]. The following is a summary of screening tools which are freely available. Tools were only included where data were available from stroke population studies, and where validity was assessed against the reference tests of FEES or VFS.

Recommended swallow screens that met these criteria were:

- 3-oz or 50ml Water Swallow Test [28-31],
- Gugging Swallow Screen (GUSS) [32]

Table 1 details the psychometric information available for these screening tools. The sensitivity measures indicate the ability of the tool to detect 'risk' when it is present, while specificity indicates the tool's ability to produce negative results for patients who are not 'at risk' [27].

A simple pulse oximetry test, in conjunction with 50ml Water Swallow Test, is reported to increase sensitivity and specificity, [28, 30] as detailed in Table 2.

Table 1. Psychometric properties of available swallow screening tools

Test	First author, year	Sensitivity %	Specificity %	PPV %	NPV %	Reference test	Reliability tested	Stroke sample size
50ml (3 oz) Water Swallow test	DePippo et al [29]	76	59			VFS	No	20
	Lim et al [30]	84.6	75	78.6	81.8	FEES	No	50
	Chong et al [28]	79.4	62.5	81.8	58.8	FEES	No	50
	Suiter & Leder [31]	92.7 - 100	40.7 – 54.8	28.4 – 33.3	95.7 - 100	FEES	No	468
Gugging Swallowing Screen (GUSS)	Trapl et al [32]	100	50 - 69	74 - 81	100	FEES	IRR between therapists (K=0.835; P<0.001)	50

PPV %= Positive predictive value; NPV %= Negative predictive value; IRR= Inter-rater reliability.

Table 2. Psychometric properties of oxygen saturation tests to detect dysphagia

Test	First author, year	Sensitivity %	Specificity %	Positive predictive value %	Negative predictive value %	Reference test	Stroke sample size
Pulse oximetry (desaturation ≥ 2%)	Lim et al [30]	76.9	83.3	83.3	76.9	FEES	50
	Chong et al [28]	55.9	100	100	51.6	FEES	50
Combined 50ml water swallow + pulse oximetry (desaturation ≥ 2%)	Lim et al [30]	100	70.8	78.8	100	FEES	50
	Chong et al [28]	94.1	62.5	84.2	83.3	FEES	50

Table 3. Swallow screens and assessments not meeting inclusion criteria

Test	First author, year	Sensitivity%	Specificity%	PPV %	NPV %	Reason for exclusion
Any Two test	Daniels et al [33]	92	67			Expert interpretation of findings needed
	Leder et al, 2002 [16]	86	30	50	73	Expert interpretation of findings needed
Bedside Swallow Assessment (BSA)	Smithard et al [21, 34]	47 –70	66 - 86	50	85	Expert interpretation of findings needed
Burke Dysphagia Screening Test (BDST)	DePippo, [35]	88	22			Only validated against pneumonia as reference test. Incorporates 3oz water swallow test which is validated.
Examination Ability to Swallow (EATS)	Courtney & Flier [36]					No validation data available
Mann Assessment of Swallowing Ability (MASA)	Mann et al [37]	73	89			Expert interpretation of findings needed
Massey Bedside Swallowing Screen	Massey & Jedlicka [38]	100	100			Only validated against clinical records of dysphagia symptoms as reference test.

Test	First author, year	Sensitivity%	Specificity%	PPV %	NPV %	Reason for exclusion
Nursing Admission Dysphagia Screening Assessment	Bravata et al [39]	29	84	50	68	Only validated against NIH Stroke Score as reference test.
Royal Brisbane & Women's Hospital Dysphagia Screening Tool	Cicherio, 2009 [12]	95	97	92	98	Only validated against SP bedside assessment
Standardised Swallow Assessment (SSA)	Ellul, 1993 [40]					No published validation data
	Perry, 2001 [27]	97	90			Only validated against 'Summative clinical judgement' as reference test
Timed Test	Hinds, 1998 [41]	97	69			Only validated against SP assessment & symptoms questionnaire as reference tests.
Toronto Bedside Swallow Screening Test (TOR-BSST)	Martino et al [6]	96	64		93	Not freely available at time of publication
Water Swallow Test (WST) - voice change finding	Nishiwaki et al [42]	72	67			Expert interpretation of findings needed

PPV%= Positive predictive value; NPV%= Negative predictive value.

The swallow assessment or screening tools which were excluded from our recommendations are detailed in Table 3. The majority of exclusions (seven tools) were due to insufficient validation of the tool, four were considered to require expert interpretation of findings and were therefore unsuitable for inter-disciplinary screening, and one tool was not freely available. Despite these short comings, this information provides a comprehensive over-view of published resources.

Swallow Screening for all?

Current stroke clinical guidelines recommend swallow screening or assessment for all patients with acute stroke. The authors' recent systematic review reported on 25 studies which examined the quality of care provided for patients with dysphagia in acute stroke settings [13]. The majority of these studies [21] included swallow screening as a process indicator of quality. Studies frequently reported poor compliance with the administration of swallow screening, which varied between settings for unclear reasons. To illustrate, Reeves et al (2008) [43] reported that only 55.6% of patients across 857 United States hospitals with an acute stroke had received a screen. By comparison the national audit of 96 Australian hospitals reported that 64% of patients were screened within 24hours of admission [5]. Rudd et al (2007) [44] described differing compliance across 46 United Kingdom hospitals depending on access to stroke unit care (73% compliance) or no stroke unit (66% compliance).

Minimal investigations have been undertaken to explore the reasons why some patients receive evidence-based care such as swallow screening, while others do not. Current evidence suggests that multiple factors contribute to the provision of quality care, including the structures and systems within health care facilities, such as stroke unit care [44, 45]. However the provision of swallow screening may also be influenced by demographic and stroke-related variables of the patients themselves, such age, gender and stroke severity. Before quality improvement activities can target barriers to care, a better understanding is needed of which patients are at risk of suboptimal care.

A Study of Swallow Screening Compliance

A recent study by the authors explored the determinants of quality care for acute stroke patients [46, 47]. One of the indicators of quality care in this study was that patients received a swallow screen within 24 hours of admission to hospital.

Methodology

Ethical approval was gained to conduct a retrospective clinical audit of consecutively sampled acute stroke patients' medical records.

Sample Size

Three hundred medical records were sampled, 100 each from three large metropolitan tertiary hospitals in Adelaide, South Australia, Australia. This sample size was sufficiently powered at $\alpha=0.05$, $\beta=0.8$ for sub-group analysis.

Inclusion and Exclusion Criteria

Patients' medical records were included if they had been consecutively admitted prior to August 31st 2009 with an IDC10 diagnostic code of acute stroke which was confirmed by diagnostic imaging or clinical evidence.

Quality of Care Measures

In an earlier systematic review we determined that *swallow screening performed within 24 hours of admission* was one appropriate measure of quality of care provided in acute stroke settings [13]. Compliance with this process indicator became the dependent variable for our investigation into the factors which influence care quality for patients with stroke related dysphagia.

Data

Data were extracted from patient records on the independent predictor variables of patients' age, gender, pre-morbid levels of independence and accommodation type, English proficiency, comorbidity levels (Charlson Comorbidity Index), weekend or weekday admission, stroke unit admission, initial stroke severity (NIH Stroke Scale), length of stay in the acute hospital (LOS), and process indicator compliance. De-identified data from all patient records were manually extracted and entered onto a purpose built MS Excel spreadsheet.

Data Analysis

We undertook a series of analyses using univariate logistic regression models to understand the relationships between the predictor variables and compliance with swallow screening. Details of this analysis, and the way that data were managed, are available elsewhere [46, 47]. Correlations between variables were expressed as odds ratios (OR) and 95% confidence intervals (95% CI).

Results

Description of Participants

The mean age of the 300 sampled patients at hospital admission was 74.7 years (Standard Deviation (SD) 13.5, range 18–100 years). The sample was proportionally balanced for gender. The mean (SD) ages for males and females were similar, however a larger proportion of females were in the older age groups with 72% females aged 75 years or older, compared to 53% males. A greater proportion of females suffered a moderate or severe stroke (28%) than males (18%). For the whole sample, there were weak relationships between increasing age and higher comorbidity levels ($r^2 = 0.20$), and increasing stroke severity ($r^2 = 0.21$). The mean length of stay in acute care was 12.5 days (SD 15.6, range 1–98 days).

Table 4. Univariate model of independent predictor variables and swallow screening

Predictor variables	Screening compliance
Age (75+ yrs)	1.02 (0.63 – 1.66)
Gender (female)	0.75 (0.47 – 1.21)
Mild stroke severity (NIHSS≤8)	*0.37 (0.23 – 0.61)**
High comorbidity (CCI ≥1)	1.29 (0.77 – 2.15)
Previous Independence	0.90 (0.54 – 1.49)
Previous residential care	1.52 (0.73 – 3.17)
Stroke unit admission	0.99 (0.62 – 1.60)
Weekend admission	*3.09 (1.84 – 5.22)**
Length of stay (<12 days)	*0.50 (0.30 – 0.82)**
English proficient	1.31 (0.54 – 3.13)
Odds Ratios (95% CIs) ** significant	

Process Indicator Compliance

Compliance with the process indicator was poor, with only 51.6% of eligible patients receiving a swallow screen within 24hrs of admission.

Variables Associated with Swallow Screening Compliance

Univariate logistic regression modelling determined that three of the 10 predictor variables were significantly associated with swallow screening compliance (see Table 4).

Patients with a mild stroke (NIHSS ≤ 8) or a shorter LOS (< 12days) were less likely to be screened than patients with more severe strokes, or those with shorter hospital stays. Swallow screens were significantly more likely to occur for patients admitted on a weekday compared to weekend admissions.

Accounting for Confounders

Additional univariate analysis demonstrated complex and potentially confounding statistical relationships between several predictor variables [47]. This is depicted in Figure 1.

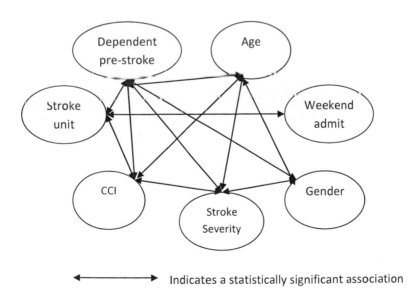

Figure 1. Potentially confounding relationships between predictor variables.

Logistical stepwise multivariate models were used to account for confounders. Only two variables were significantly associated with the provision of swallow screening, after confounders were considered in analysis (Table 5).

Table 5. Variables associated with swallow screening after accounting for confounders

Predictor variables	Screening compliance	
	Chi^2 [Freedom°]	OR (95% CI)
Mild stroke severity (NIHSS≤8)	16.2 [1]	*0.4 (0.2-0.6)* **
Length of stay (<12 days)	19.0 [2]	0.6 (0.4-1.1)
Weekend admission	36.1 [2]	*3.3 (1.9-5.7)* **

** Statistically significant finding OR= Odds ratio.
95%CI= 95% Confidence Interval.

Discussion of Study Findings

This study provides new findings regarding the factors which may relate to compliance with swallow screening for acute stroke patients. Our findings support earlier studies reporting the sub-optimal use of swallow screening in practice. The complex associations identified between independent variables indicate that there are unlikely to be simple explanations for why some patients receive recommended dysphagia care and others do not.

We acknowledge that the generalizability of the findings may be limited by some variables chosen in our study, due to international variations in health care policy and systems. Length of stay data and admissions directly to a stroke unit, for example, are both particularly influenced by local contexts.

Our results indicate that patients admitted over a weekend or with mild strokes (NIHSS scores ≤8) may be at particular risk of missing swallow screening. Previous studies have also reported poor quality care for patients admitted over weekends, and have linked this to worse outcomes for these patients [44, 48]. The reasons for day-dependent differences in care standards are unclear but are likely to be associated with the reduced availability of trained staff and different operational systems over weekends. It appears that staff are mindful of performing a swallow screen for patients admitted with a severe stroke, perhaps due to more visible cues of risk. However there is no evidence that patients with milder strokes (as determined by NIHSS) are at less risk of dysphagia than patients who have had a more severe stroke. The recommendation of swallow screening for all stroke admissions needs to be more universally implemented.

Improving Compliance
with Swallow Screening

The principles of translating evidence into clinical practice have been well documented by implementation scientists in recent years [49-51]. Strategies specific to clinical management in acute stroke settings are emerging and could be applied to the improvement of effective swallow screen processes [11, 12, 52-55]. Evidence based strategies that could be considered include: organisational assessment of readiness for practice change, identification of barriers to change, effective involvement of key stakeholders, development of incentives to change, targeted education programs, and the guided roll-out of the new practices followed by cycles of clinical auditing and feedback.

The research outlined above suggests that there are particular sub-groups of acute stroke patients who may be at increased risk of poor dysphagia management. The swallow screening implementation strategies should ensure that these at-risk groups are carefully considered.

Conclusion

Dysphagia is a common consequence of stroke that must be identified early after onset and managed carefully to avoid negative outcomes. Swallow screening for all acute stroke patients is recommended best-practice to efficiently detect those patients at risk of swallowing problems. Debate continues regarding the best way to conduct screening. This chapter identified two swallow screening tools that have proven sensitivity and specificity in the acute stroke population. Both these tools can be used by staff from various disciplines, after minimal training.

The effective application of swallow screening within clinical settings is challenging. Current evidence suggests that universal swallow screening is not well translated into clinical practice. Some patients may be at greater risk from unidentified dysphagia than others. The results of our recent study demonstrated that patients admitted over a weekend and those with milder strokes were more likely to miss out on timely swallow screening. Acute stroke facilities should consider systematic ways to ensure optimal care for all patients.

References

[1]   NSF. National Stroke Foundation Annual Review. *2010 achievements…10 years of progress… tomorrows challenge.* Melbourne Australia: National Stroke Foundation, 2010.

[2]   Senes S. *How we manage stroke in Australia.* Canberra: Australian Institute of Health and Welfare 2006.

[3]   NSF. *Clinical Guidelines for Stroke Management 2010.* Melbourne Australia: National Stroke Foundation 2010.

[4]   Pendlebury S, Rothwell P. Stroke management and prevention. *Medicine.* 2004;32:62.

[5]   National Stroke F. *National Stroke Audit Acute Services Organisational Survey Report.* Melbourne: National Stroke Foundation 2009.

[6]   Martino R, Foley N, Bhogal S, Diamant N, Speechley M, Teasell R. Dysphagia after stroke: Incidence, diagnosis and pulmonary complications. *Stroke.* 2005;36:2756.

[7]   Nilsson H, Ekberg O, Olsson R, Hindfelt B. Dysphagia in stroke: a prospective study of quantitative aspects of swallowing in dysphagic patients. *Dysphagia.* 1998;13:6.

[8]   Daniels SK, Ballo LA, Mahoney MC, Foundas AL. Clinical predictors of dysphagia and aspiration risk: Outcome measures in acute stroke patients. *Arch Phys Med Rehabil.* 2000;81(8):1030.

[9]   Foley NC, Salter KL, Robertson J, Teasell RW, Woodbury MG. Which reported estimate of the prevalence of malnutrition after stroke is valid? *Stroke.* 2009;40(3):e66.

[10] Hinchey J, Shephard T, Furie K, Smith D, Wang D, Tonn S. Formal dysphagia screening protocols prevent pneumonia. *Stroke.* 2005;36(9):1972.

[11] Perry L, McLaren S. Implementing evidence based guidelines for nutrition support in acute stroke. *Evidence Based Nursing.* 2003;6:68-71.

[12] Cichero JA, Heaton S, Bassett L. Triaging dysphagia: nurse screening for dysphagia in an acute hospital. *Journal of Clinical Nursing.* 2009;18(11):1649.

[13] Luker JA, Wall K, Bernhardt J, Edwards I, Grimmer-Somers KA. Measuring the quality of dysphagia management following stroke: a systematic review. *International Journal of Stroke.* 2010;5:466.

[14] Logemann JA. *Evaluation and Treatment of Swallowing Disorders.* 2nd ed. Austin, Texas: Pro-Ed; 1998.

[15] Weinhardt J, Hazelett S, Barrett D, Lada R, Enos T, Keleman R. Accuracy of a bedside dysphagia screening: a comparison of registered nurses and speech therapists. *Rehabilitation Nursing.* 2008;33(6):247.

[16] Leder SB, Espinosa JF, Leder SB, Espinosa JF. Aspiration risk after acute stroke: comparison of clinical examination and fiberoptic endoscopic evaluation of swallowing. *Dysphagia.* [Comparative Study]. 2002;17(3):214-8.

[17] Nakajoh K, Nakagawa T, Sekizawa K, Matsui T, Arai H, Sasaki H. Relation between incidence of pneumonia and protective reflexes in post-stroke patients with oral or tube feeding. *Journal of Internal Medicine.* 2000;247(1):4.

[18] Ramsey DJ, Smithard DG, Kalra L, Ramsey DJC, Smithard DG, Kalra L. Early assessments of dysphagia and aspiration risk in acute stroke patients. *Stroke.* 2003;34(5):1252-7.

[19] Horner J, Massey EW. Silent aspiration following stroke. Neurology. 1988;38(2):317-9.

[20] McCullough GH, Wertz RT, Rosenbek JC. Sensitivity and specificity of clinical/bedside examination signs for detecting aspiration in adults subsequent to stroke. *Journal of Communication Disorders.* 2001;34(1/2):55.

[21] Smithard DG, O'Neill PA, Park C, England R, Renwick DS, Wyatt R, et al. Can bedside assessment reliably exclude aspiration following acute stroke? *Age & Ageing.* 1998;27(2):99.

[22] Daniels SK, Schroeder MF, DeGeorge PC, Corey DM, Foundas AL, Rosenbek JC. Defining and measuring dysphagia following stroke. *American Journal of Speech-Language Pathology.* 2009;18(1):74.

[23] Martin-Harris B, Brodsky MB, Michel Y, Castell DO, Schleicher M, Sandidge J, et al. MBS measurement tool for swallow impairment--MBSImp: esablishing a standard. *Dysphagia.* 2008;23(4):392.

[24] Langmore SE, Schatz K, Olson N. Endoscopic and videofluoroscopic evaluations of swallowing and aspiration. *Annals of Otology, Rhinology & Laryngology.* [Comparative Study]. 1991;100(8):678-81.

[25] Bours GJJ, Speyer R, Lemmens J, Limburg M, de Wit R. Bedside screening tests vs. videofluoroscopy or fibreoptic endoscopic evaluation of swallowing to detect dysphagia in patients with neurological disorders: systematic review. *Journal of Advanced Nursing.* 2009;65(3):477.

[26] Martino R, Pron G, Diamant N. Screening for oropharyngeal dysphagia in stroke: Insufficient evidence for guidelines. *Dysphagia.* 2000;15:19.

[27] Perry L. Screening swallowing function of patients with acute stroke. Part one: identification, implementation and initial evaluation of a screening tool for use by nurses. *Journal of Clinical Nursing.* 2001;10(4):463.

[28] Chong MS, Lieu PK, Sitoh YY, Meng YY, Leow LP. Bedside clinical methods useful as screening test for aspiration in elderly patients with recent and previous strokes. *AnnAcadMedSingap.* 2003;32(6):790.

[29] DePippo KL, Holas MA, Reding MJ. Validation of the 3-oz water swallow test for aspiration following stroke. *Archives of Neurology.* 1992;49(12):1259.

[30] Lim S, Lieu P, Phua S, Seshadri R, Venketasubramanian N, Lee S, et al. Accuracy of bedside clinical methods compared to fiberoptic endoscopic examination of swallow (FEES) in determining the risk of aspiration in acute stroke patients. *Dysphagia.* 2001;16(1):1.

[31] Suiter DM, Leder SB. Clinical utility of the 3-ounce water swallow test. *Dysphagia.* 2008;23(3):244.

[32] Trapl M, Enderle P, Nowotny M, Teuschl Y, Matz K, Dachenhausen A, et al. Dysphagia bedside screening for acute-stroke patients: the Gugging Swallowing Screen. *Stroke.* 2007;38(11):2948.

[33] Daniels SK, McAdam CP, Brailey K, Foundas AL. Clinical assessment of swallowing and prediction of dysphagia severity. *American Journal of Speech-Language Pathology.* 1997;6:17.

[34] Smithard DG, O'Neill PA, Park C, Morris J, Wyatt R, England R, et al. Complications and Outcome After Acute Stroke: Does Dysphagia Matter? *Stroke.* 1996;27(7):1200.

[35] DePippo KL, Holas MA, Reding MJ. The Burke dysphagia screening test: validation of its use in patients with stroke. *Archives of Physical Medicine & Rehabilitation.* 1994;75(12):1284.

[36] Courtney BA, Flier LA. RN dysphagia screening, a stepwise approach. *Journal of Neuroscience Nursing.* 2009;41(1):28.

[37] Man DWK, Tam SF, Hui-Chan CWY. Learning to live independently with expert systems in memory rehabilitation. *NeuroRehabilitation.* 2002;18(1):21.

[38] Massey R, Jedlicka D. The Massey Bedside Swallowing Screen. *Journal of Neuroscience Nursing.* 2002;34(5):252.

[39] Bravata DM, Daggett VS, Woodward-Hagg H, Damush T, Plue L, Russell S, et al. Comparison of two approaches to screen for dysphagia among acute ischemic stroke patients: nursing admission screening tool versus National Institutes of Health stroke scale. *Journal of Rehabilitation Research & Development.* 2009;46(9):1127.

[40] Ellul J, Barer D, Group NWDS. Detection and management of dysphagia in patients with acute stroke. *Age & Ageing*. 1993;22(Suppl 2)(17).

[41] Hinds NP, Wiles CM. Assessment of swallowing and referral to speech and language therapists in acute stroke. *QJM*. 1998;91(12):829-35.

[42] Nishiwaki K, Tsuji T, Liu M, Hase K, Tanaka N, Fujiwara T. Identification of a simple screening tool for dysphagia in patients with stroke using factor analysis of multiple dysphagia variables. Journal *of Rehabilitation Medicine*. 2005;37(4):247.

[43] Reeves MJ, Smith E, Fonarow G, Hernandez A, Pan W, Schwamm LH, et al. Off-hour admission and in-hospital stroke case fatality in the get with the guidelines-stroke program. *Stroke*. 2009;40(2):569.

[44] Rudd AG, Hoffman A, Down C, Pearson M, Lowe D. Access to stroke care in England, Wales and Northern Ireland: the effect of age, gender and weekend admission. *Age & Ageing*. 2007;36(3):247.

[45] Lingsma HF, Dippel DW, Hoeks SE, Steyerberg EW, Franke CL, van Oostenbrugge RJ, et al. Variation between hospitals in patient outcome after stroke is only partly explained by differences in quality of care: results from the Netherlands Stroke Survey. *Journal of Neurology, Neurosurgery & Psychiatry*. 2008;79(8):888.

[46] Luker JA, Bernhardt J, Grimmer-Somers KA. Age and gender as predictors of allied health quality stroke care. *J Multidiscip Healthc*. 2011;4:1.

[47] Luker JA, Bernhardt J, Grimmer-Somers KA. Demographic and stroke-related factors as predictors of quality of acute stroke care provided by allied health professionals. *J Multidiscip Healthc*. 2011;4.

[48] Saposnik G, Baibergenova A, Bayer N, Hachinski V. Weekends: a dangerous time for having a stroke? see comment. Stroke. 2007;38(4):1211.

[49] Grol R, Buchan H. Clinical guidelines: what can we do to increase their use? *Medical Journal of Australia*. 2006;185(6):301.

[50] Grimshaw J, Eccles M. Is evidence-based implementation of evidence-based care possible? Medical Journal of Australia. 2004;180:S50.

[51] Grol R, Wensing M. What drives change? Barriers to and incentives for achieving evidence-based practice. *Medical Journal of Australia*. 2004;180:S57.

[52] Perry L. Promoting evidence-based practice in stroke care in Australia. *Nursing Standard*. 2006;20(34):35.

[53] Gropen T, Magdon-Ismail Z, Day D, Melluzzo S, Schwamm LH. Regional implementation of the stroke systems of care model: Recommendations of the northeast cerebrovascular consortium. *Stroke*. 2009;40(5):1793.

[54] Stoeckle-Roberts S, Reeves MJ, Jacobs BS, Maddox K, Choate L, Wehner S, et al. Closing gaps between evidence-based stroke care guidelines and practices with a collaborative quality improvement project. *Joint Commission Journal on Quality & Patient Safety.* 2006;32(9):517.

[55] Pollock A, Legg L, Langhorne P, Sellars C. Barriers to achieving evidence-based stroke rehabilitation. *Clinical Rehabilitation.* 2000;14(6):611.

In: Dysphagia   ISBN 978-1-61942-104-2
Editors: B. S. Smith and M. Adams   © 2012 Nova Science Publishers, Inc.

Chapter V

Dysphagia: Perioperative Risk Factors, Diagnosis and Treatment

P. Bradley Segebarth and Bruce Darden
OrthoCarolina Spine Center, Charlotte, North Carolina, US

Abstract

Swallowing disorders are a significant cause of morbidity and mortality. Unrecognized dysphagia can lead to dehydration, malnutrition, aspiration pneumonia, or airway difficulty. The etiology is numerous and may be neurologic, muscular, or obstructive. Though many conditions may be associated with dysphagia, iatrogenic causes are also common. Anterior cervical spine surgery is often associated with varying degrees of post-operative swallowing difficulties. Understanding the risk factors as well as the anatomy and pathophysiology of swallowing should aid diagnosis, treatment, and limitation of dysphagia complications.

After identifying there is a swallowing problem, the anatomic region or involved phase should be recognized. History alone may be enough to detect an esophageal etiology, but oral and pharyngeal phase problems are best delineated by careful physical exam and diagnosis often aided by radiographic and laboratory studies. Once cause is identified, treatment is individualized based on structural and functional abnormalities. If underlying cause of dysphagia is not treatable, a combination of dietary modifications and swallowing therapy is often helpful. In some patients, enteral therapy may be necessary in the short term or long term in extreme cases in order to provide adequate nutrition.

Introduction

Dysphagia is a well-known complication following anterior cervical discectomy and fusion. Reported frequency ranges widely in various reported studies [3,27,14]. A recent systematic review notes an incidence range from 1% to 79% within one week of surgery, declining to 13% to 21% at one year after operation [28]. The etiology is likely multifactorial and has been attributed to hematoma, pharyngeal plexus denervation, vocal cord paresis, adhesion formation, plate profile, and swelling due to biologic agents [3,14,34,19,32]. Severe cases of dysphagia can lead to significant morbidity and mortality, including dehydration, malnutrition, aspiration pneumonia, and airway difficulty. This chapter will aim to identify risk factors, enhance diagnosis, and provide treatment recommendations for post-operative swallowing difficulties. Additionally, a better understanding of the pathophysiology may help minimize dysphagia complications by utilizing preventative measures intra-operatively.

Anatomy and Physiology of Swallowing

The act of swallowing is a complex coordination of events involving the mouth, pharynx, larynx, and esophagus. The ability to close the respiratory tract from the alimentary tract involves coordinated central neural control. The swallowing center in the brainstem is adjacent to sensory and motor nuclei of the vagus nerve and is near the area that controls respiration [5]. This area of the brainstem relays the glottic closure reflex. Coordination of pharyngeal function during swallowing is orchestrated by the pharyngeal plexus, consisting of the glossopharyngeal nerve and the pharyngeal branch of the vagus nerve. Anterior cervical exposure above the level of C3 may put at risk the hypoglossal or glossopharyngeal nerves, while the mid cervical levels impart more risk to other nerves of the pharyngeal plexus [17].

The vagus nerve provides motor and sensory function to the palate, pharynx, esophagus, stomach, and respiratory tract. It travels in the carotid sheath adjacent the internal carotid and then common carotid artery as it descends the neck, giving off several important branches. The superior laryngeal nerve comes off the vagus high in the neck and gives rise to internal and external branches [5]. One cadaveric study describes the course of the external superior laryngeal nerve as being variable, but safe from anterior cervical spine dissection above the level of c3-4 and below c6-7. In this study, the internal branch of the superior laryngeal nerve was consistently exposed within one centimeter of the c3-4 disc space. The external branch was found deep to the superior thyroid artery, the origin of which was found most commonly located at the c4 level. The external superior laryngeal nerve was found to be less bulky and more taut than the internal branch [17]. In terms of function, the external branch innervates the cricothyroid muscle, which tenses the vocal cord and aids in ability to produce high notes. The internal branch of the superior laryngeal nerve provides sensation to the supraglottic region and hypopharynx, and is therefore critical in protecting against aspiration.

The recurrent laryngeal nerve also originates from the vagus nerve. On the right, it loops around the right subclavian artery and then crosses the anterolateral cervical spine in a circuitous cephalad path before entering the tracheoesophageal groove. The left recurrent laryngeal nerve originates where the vagus nerve crosses the aortic arch, loops under the ligamentum arteriosum, and travels cephalad in the tracheoesophageal groove more medial and predictably than on the right. For this reason, the left-sided approach to the cervical spine may potentially have less risk of stretch injury to the recurrent laryngeal nerve than a right-sided approach [33]. The recurrent laryngeal nerve supplies sensation to the glottic and subglottic regions as well as motor to all of the intrinsic laryngeal muscles except the cricothyroid muscle, which is supplied directly by the vagus. The cricoarytenoid muscles, supplied by the recurrent laryngeal nerves, are the only muscles that abduct the vocal cords. (image 1)

The act of swallowing is divided into three phases: oral, pharyngeal, and esophageal. The oral phase is under voluntary control and involves the lips, tongue, mandible, palate, and cheeks acting together to grind and deliver food to the pharynx. This function relies in large part on the cranial nerves, including the trigeminal, glossopharyngeal, facial, hypoglossal, as well as the vagus nerves. The coordination of the soft palate, peristalsis of the tongue, salivary glands, and facial muscles are a result of both chemo and chechanoreceptors in the mouth that interchange information between facial, glossopharyngeal, and hypoglossal nerves [19].

The pharyngeal phase begins when the leading edge of food bolus passes posterior to the faucial arch. This initiates an involuntary coordination of muscle contractions that include laryngeal elevation and inversion of the epiglottis and closure of the true and false vocal folds. The soft palate closes to prevent reflux. The larynx closes to prevent aspiration. The pharyngeal constrictor muscles move the bolus, and the cricopharyngeus muscle relaxes to allow food to pass into the esophagus. This phase is primarily mediated by the internal branch of the superior laryngeal nerve, along with glossopharyngeal and recurrent laryngeal nerves at the lower larynx level [5].

The final phase of swallowing is the involuntary esophageal phase. The upper third of the esophagus consists of striated muscle, middle third striated and smooth muscle, and the lower third smooth muscle. These layers propagate peristaltic waves transferring food boluses into the stomach. The neural coordination of this peristalsis occurs through the autonomic myenteric plexus of Auerbach, located between the longitudinal and circular muscle layers in the esophagus. This plexus is triggered by the vagus nerve [19].

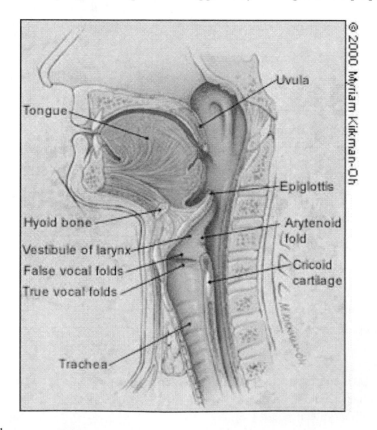

Image 1.

Aspiration prevention is mediated by both basal and response mechanisms. The vagus nerve mediates upper and lower esophageal sphincter control, giving basal mechanism of aspiration prevention. Response mechanisms include esophagoglottal reflex, pharyngoglottal closure reflex, pharyngo-upper esophagus reflex, and the esophago-upper esophagus reflex. These act in response to mechanical stimulation of the pharynx or distension of the esophagus [5,23].

Swallowing Disorders

Post-operative dysphagia can be categorized according to the swallowing phase that is affected, and particular dysfunction patterns can suggest the underlying etiology. After anterior cervical surgery, injury to related structures most often affects the oral and pharyngeal phases of swallowing. Less commonly, problems with esophageal phase of swallowing result in retention of food and liquid in the esophagus resulting from a motility dysfunction or impaired opening of the lower esophageal sphincter.

Problems with the oral preparatory phase often result from impaired control of the tongue, suggesting injury to the hypoglossal or glossopharyngeal nerves. With solid food, the patient may experience difficulty chewing and initiating swallows. When drinking, it may be difficult to contain the liquid in the oral cavity before swallowing. This could result in liquid spilling into the unprepared pharynx, and result in aspiration.

Pharyngeal phase dysfunction affects food transport to the esophagus, leaving retained food or liquid in the pharynx after swallowing. Though small amounts of food are commonly retained in the valleculae or pyriform sinus with normal swallowing, excessive retention can result in overflow aspiration. This can be the result of weakness or incoordination of the pharyngeal muscles or poor opening of the upper esophageal sphincter [16].

Videofluoroscopic studies have been utilized to analyze patterns of swallowing abnormalities after surgery. One such study found a variety of dysphagia patterns in all stages of swallowing. Some had absent pharyngeal swallow pattern consistent with superior laryngeal nerve injury, others demonstrated oral preparatory phase impairment with inferred damage to the hypoglossal nerve. Still other patterns were consistent with prevertebral soft tissue swelling causing reduced pharyngeal wall movement, impaired upper esophageal opening, incomplete epiglottic deflection, and incomplete pharyngeal emptying with retained residue [21].

Aspiration is a serious clinical complication resulting from post-operative dysphagia which involves passage of food or liquid through the vocal folds. This is often caused by impaired laryngeal closure or overflow of food or liquid retained in the pharynx. It increases risk for other respiratory problems such as airway obstruction and aspiration pneumonia. Though microscopic aspiration is normal and can be well tolerated, gross aspiration of larger quantities poses more risk and can involve the distal airways. Normal pulmonary clearance mechanisms may also be affected. If sensation is impaired, the strong cough reflex may be absent and silent aspiration results without cough or throat clearing. The content of material aspirated also plays a role. Solid food may cause frank airway obstruction, while acidic material is highly caustic to the lung parenchyma. Aspirating material containing infectious organisms or even normal mouth flora can cause bacterial pneumonitis.

Incidence and Risk Factors

Though frequently reported as a common complication after anterior cervical spine surgery, the published incidence of dysphagia varies widely. Several factors likely contribute to this variance. Most studies on this subject are retrospective, relying on medical records rather than patient surveys to track dysphagia. This method has been shown to underreport complications [12]. Additionally, there is no universally accepted definition or method of determining the presence of dysphagia after surgery. Though radiographic tests such as videofluoroscopy can be accurate in detecting swallowing abnormalities, their utilization as a screening tool for postoperative swallowing problems is questionable. Patient-reported outcomes have been shown to be reliable and valid, and are preferred over clinician-reported outcomes or a physiologic study [10]. Though seemingly underutilized, two outcome questionnaires have been determined to be valid and reliable: the MD Anderson Dysphagia Inventory, and the "Difficulty Swallowing" portion of the Cervical Spine Outcomes Questionnaire [7,4]. (image 2)

Despite the variable reported incidence, a common theme in the literature is that the prevalence of postoperative dysphagia decreases over time [3]. A recent systematic review on postoperative dysphagia compares fourteen prospective and one registry study to summarize the best available evidence on the subject. Dysphagia rates after anterior cervical discectomy and fusion ranged from 1-79% within one week of surgery, 50-56% one month after surgery, 8-22% at six months, and 13-21% one year after surgery [28]. In addition to anterior cervical discectomy and fusion surgery, other anterior cervical procedures also show increased risk of postoperative dysphagia. In one series reported on anterior osteosynthesis for odontoid fractures in the elderly, 35% of patients required diet modification or nasogastric tube after surgery due to swallowing difficulties 9).

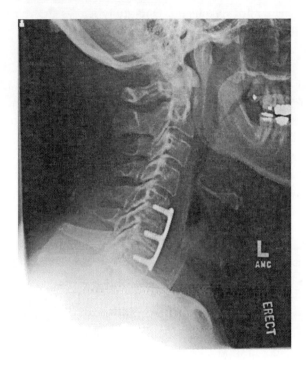

Image 2.

The etiology of postoperative dysphagia is multifactorial, and has been attributed to hematoma, pharyngeal plexus denervation, vocal cord paralysis, adhesion formation, plate profile, and swelling due to biologic agents [3,14,34,20,32. Risk factors proposed include female gender, age>60, multi-level surgery, revision surgery, and length of surgery. Of these, only female gender and multilevel surgery met criteria for "moderate" supporting evidence according to Riley et al. [28].

Aside from the factors introduced at the time of surgery, some patients may be at more risk for postoperative dysphagia due to baseline medical problems. Underlying neurologic disorders can predispose to swallowing difficulties and may include conditions such as prior stroke, parkinson's, multiple sclerosis, myasthenia gravis, poliomyelitis, amyotrophic lateral sclerosis, and dementia. Connective tissue disorders such as polymyositis and muscular dystrophy may also be at more risk for dysphagia. Other medical treatments which may exacerbate dysphagia include psychotropic medications, prior radiation, or previous neck surgery.

Even the underlying spinal condition for which surgery is being performed may be a risk factor for dysphagia. One study shows that posterior cervical surgery had a higher incidence of dysphagia than lumbar surgery controls, yet not as high of incidence as anterior cervical surgery [30].

Another study showed that the risk of developing postoperative dysphagia increases with time since the first episode of pain [27]. An additional study demonstrated approximately 50% of patients undergoing anterior cervical surgery had evidence of preoperative swallowing abnormalities without an underlying medical cause [15]. Possible explanations of these findings include decreased sensitivity of pharyngeal and supraglottic areas with aging, or underlying cervical spondylosis interfering with preganglionic sympathetic outflow or the spinal afferent nerves.

Interestingly, some evidence suggests that motion-sparing anterior cervical surgeries may have a lower incidence of postoperative dysphagia. Three separate studies utilizing different arthroplasty devices show decreased dysphagia rates after surgery compared to anterior cervical discectomy and fusion groups [1,22,30]. This may be due to lack of hardware in the anterior retropharyngeal space or continued motion at the operative site. More studies involving newer technologies such as cervical disc arthroplasty and stand-alone plate-spacer devices are needed in order to draw any solid conclusions regarding risk factors for postoperative dysphagia.

Prevention

Though the evidence is limited, some studies suggest changing operative techniques or implants may positively influence the incidence of postoperative dysphagia after anterior cervical surgery. Apfelbaum et al. hypothesized pressure-related damage to the recurrent laryngeal nerve from the inflated endotracheal tube cuff and the anterior cervical retractors. A cadaveric study supported the fact that cuff pressures greatly increased after retractor placement [2,18]. By releasing and then re-inflating the cuff after retractor placement, the endotracheal tube was allowed a more central position within the larynx. Using this maneuver in 650 anterior procedures, the rate of recurrent laryngeal palsy fell from 6.8% to 1.7%. Another study monitoring intra-operative endotracheal cuff pressures showed that adjusting the cuff pressure to about 20 mm Hg and minimizing retraction time correlated with lower sore throat, hoarseness, and dysphagia up to 24 hours after surgery [26]. However, one week after surgery there was no significant difference between the two groups.

Several studies focus on the plate design or anterior profile as it relates to postoperative dysphagia after anterior cervical surgery. One report compared a thicker and wider plate to a smaller and smoother plate in 156 consecutive patients undergoing anterior cervical discectomy and fusion [20]. At six months, the smaller and smoother plate had a lower incidence of patient-reported dysphagia (14% vs. 22.5%). This trend continued out to one year follow up and became statistically significant at two year follow up with no patients in the smaller plate group reporting ongoing dysphagia. However, a recent prospective study questions the role of plate thickness as a cause of dysphagia [8]. In contrast to prior studies [31,3,20,27], the cervical plating study sponsored by the Cervical Spine Research Society (CSRS) comparing instrumented and uninstrumented ACDF patients showed a slight increase in the incidence of dysphagia with anterior instrumentation of 7.9% vs. 5.3% in the uninstrumented group at 24 months follow-up.

In addition to plate prominence, adhesion formation to esophageal and pharyngeal structures may play a role in postoperative dysphagia. One recent study involved anatomic mapping of the esophagus and vertebral bodies to help determine the effect of plate profile on surrounding structures [29]. Fogel et al. reported on the surgical exploration and removal of anterior hardware for persistent moderate to severe dysphagia symptoms [13]. Intraoperative findings for all patients demonstrated significant adhesions of the pharynx and esophagus to the plate by scar, which was released before plate removal. Fifty-five percent of patients had resolution of their dysphagia and an additional 32% reported dysphagia improvement to mild symptoms.

Anterior cervical disc arthroplasty outcomes have been compared to anterior cervical discectomy and fusion. Three studies utilizing three different arthroplasty devices have shown lower incidence of post-operative dysphagia compared to the fusion groups [1,22,30].

Theoretically, this could be due in part to implant profile or preservation of motion leading to less adhesions. However, no strong conclusions can be drawn with regards to postoperative dysphagia risks with arthroplasty, and further studies would be helpful.

Despite the literature cited above, there is very low evidence that intraoperative reduction of entotracheal cuff pressure or plate design have any effect on the rate of postoperative dysphagia [28]. Additionally, methylprednisolone as a means to decrease postoperative swelling has not been shown to effect dysphagia rates [25].

It stands to reason that knowing the anatomy and structures at risk for injury may help to prevent iatrogenic causes of postoperative dysphagia after anterior cervical surgery. Meticulous dissection and hemostasis to minimize scar formation, and limiting retraction time should decrease traction injury to neural and muscular structures.

Evaluation

As with any condition in medicine, a thorough history is of utmost importance in identifying those at risk for postoperative dysphagia. Medications should be reviewed, as a number of psychotropic drugs can exacerbate swallowing difficulties. A history of stroke or other underlying neurological disorders such as Parkinson's disease or dementia may effect swallowing function. Gastroesophageal reflux disease, diabetes, prior neck radiation or surgery all increase risk of swallowing problems after surgery, even if the patient is asymptomatic preoperatively. One should strongly consider an otolaryngology evaluation in any patient with a prior history of hoarseness, voice change, and in those patients undergoing revision surgery. A laryngoscopic exam is particularly important when planning a unilateral approach on the opposite side from a prior anterior cervical surgery, to rule out subclinical injury to the superior laryngeal or recurrent laryngeal nerves.

Whether evaluating preoperatively or after anterior cervical surgery, it is important to identify the anatomic region involved with swallowing difficulty. The oral and pharyngeal phases can give symptoms of choking, coughing, drooling, voice change, difficulty initiating swallowing, and symptoms of food sticking to the throat. An esophageal etiology might give symptoms of food sticking in the chest, heartburn, belching, and regurgitation.

On inspection, neck swelling or palpable masses should be noted. Abnormal voice or speech articulation may indicate motor dysfunction to structures in the oral and pharyngeal swallowing phases. Laryngeal elevation can be assessed by placing two fingers on the larynx and checking movement during volitional swallowing. Any asymmetry of the soft palate during phonation and rest should be noted. A gag reflex is checked by stroking the pharyngeal mucosa with a cotton-tipped applicator. If the palate pulls to one side during gag reflex, this indicates weakness of the contralateral palate suggesting unilateral brain-stem pathology [24].

The patient should be observed swallowing a few ounces of tap water. This is an important test postoperatively to evaluate for any signs or symptoms of moderate or severe dysphagia. Normally, swallowing is initiated promptly, and no significant amount of material is retained. Drooling, delayed swallowing initiation, coughing, throat clearing, or a change of voice may indicate a problem. After the swallow, assess for any delayed cough response. If the water swallow test is abnormal, further testing is warranted prior to advancing feeds.

A speech pathologist should be consulted postoperatively if there is any concern for swallowing problems that may effect feeding regimen. A bedside swallow study would include the water swallow test and assessment of swallowing pattern. A videofluorographic swallowing study can better assess the mechanism of swallowing. The patient is seated and given a mixture of food and drink mixed with radiopaque barium. Videofluoroscopy demonstrates the motions of the anatomic structures as the barium bolus is passed through the oral cavity, pharynx, and esophagus. If present, aspiration is noted and quantified. Any retention of food or liquid is noted, as well as the patient's response to retention or aspiration.

By testing various food consistencies, the videofluoroscopy study allows the therapist to design an individualized diet. Patients with poor bolus control often experience less aspiration with thick liquids such as nector. Those with poor pharyngeal contraction usually have more pharyngeal retention with thickened liquids and solid foods than with thin liquids. Compensatory mechanisms can be tested to determine what the patient is safely capable of swallowing. Tucking the chin or holding the breath before swallowing may reduce aspiration. Turning the head toward the weak side may improve pharyngeal clearance. If a videofluoroscopic exam is not feasible, a fiberoptic endoscopic exam may be an alternative. However, if patient unable to participate in volitional swallowing safely, parenteral nutrition should be considered.

Treatment

The treatment for postoperative dysphagia should be based on specific mechanism of dysfunction. Given that most swallowing problems after anterior cervical surgery predictably improve with time, treatments often serve as a temporary bridge until swallowing improves. Nevertheless, the early postoperative period is both a critical time for patient nutrition as well as a period of particular risk for dysphagia complications and their sequelae. The goals of therapy are to reduce aspiration, improve ability to eat, and optimize nutritional status. Repeat evaluations with a speech pathologist are necessary to advance diet as swallowing improves.

Once the patient has been evaluated for swallowing dysfunction and effective compensatory abilities, treatment is individualized. Dietary modification is based on ability to tolerate various food consistencies. Thin or thick liquid diet can usually provide adequate oral hydration. If these liquids are demonstrated to be an aspiration risk, a thicker pudding consistency may be necessary. Hydration can be supplemented intravenously. With patients who exhibit difficulties with the oral preparatory phase or those who have significant pharyngeal retention of chewed solid foods, a pureed diet is prescribed [24].

Swallowing therapy involves compensatory maneuvers or techniques that can be tested during videofluoroscopy. By altering the position of the head, neck and body relative to gravity the opening of the upper esophageal sphincter may be improved, increasing pharyngeal clearance and minimizing aspiration. The patient may also be taught to voluntarily contract particular muscles during the act of swallowing. Indirect therapy is also initiated to help strengthen swallowing muscles.

On rare occasion, surgery may be indicated in patients with chronic oral or pharyngeal dysphagia. A cricopharyneal myotomy may reduce resistance of pharyngeal outflow, and can be coupled with suspension of the thryrod cartilage to improve laryngeal elevation. The specific indications and contraindications remain unclear, and are best evaluated by an otolaryngologist. If retained hardware is thought to be the main contributing factor for persistent swallowing difficulties, this can be addressed surgicallyas well. Fogel demonstrated improvement of dysphagia with removal of the anterior cervical plates and release of mechanical adhesions of the esophagus. [13]

When a postoperative patient is unable to obtain adequate nutrition from the above treatments, enteral feeding is considered. Aspiration alone does not always necessitate enteral feeding. A modified diet and use of compensatory maneuvers can allow most patients with minimal aspiration and adequate clearance mechanisms to take sufficient food and drink by mouth to meet nutritional requirements. This also allows those patients to continue swallowing, thereby exercising their dysfunctional muscles. Those patients with impaired levels of consciousness, massive aspiration, silent aspiration, or recurrent respiratory infections will require enteral feedings. Periodic repeat evaluations by the speech therapist are useful for advancing diet and discontinuing enteral feedings.

When risk factors for postoperative dysphagia are significant, and nutrition in question, the authors recommend placing a nasogastric feeding tube at the time of surgery. If bedside evaluation postoperatively proves concern for adequate and safe nutrition, then the feedings may begin promptly. This also engages the patient's family and support group early so as not to alarm them with unexpected complications. In cases that prove to have persistent dysphagia interfering with nutrition, a percutaneous endoscopic gastrostomy is considered for long-term enteral nutrition. This should be discussed preoperatively as a possibility with those patients who are at greatest risk for problems.

Conclusion

Swallowing difficulties are a well known complication after anterior cervical surgery and not limited to fusions or instrumentation cases. Patients should be advised of this preoperatively, and expect some dysphagia symptoms after surgery. Those with significant risk factors should be counseled about the possible interventions that may be necessary, such as feeding tube placement. Swallowing difficulties postoperatively are generally expected to decrease over time, though a minority of patients experience some degree of persistent symptoms beyond one year postoperative [28]. For this reason, the surgeon should routinely assess for symptoms after surgery. The best self-assesment tool would include global, functional, psychosocial, and physical domains. Those patients who have severe or persistent problems may benefit from evaluation by a speech therapist to initiate appropriate exercises or therapy. Surgical planning and technique may minimize complications from stretch injury to oropharyngeal nerves. Familiarity with the anatomy and at-risk structures as well as minimizing retraction to pharyngeal musculature may decrease the incidence of dysphagia. Meticulous tissue dissection and hemostasis should theoretically help reduce scar formation and adhesions postoperatively. While the clinical evidence is weak, smoother and lower contour plates as well as deflation and re-inflation of endotracheal tube cuff may decrease the incidence of postoperative dysphagia [28]. Any patient with delayed dysphagia presentation or marked early decompensation should be evaluated clinically and radiographically for graft dislodgement, postoperative hematoma or edema, or retropharyngeal abscess.

References

[1]   Anderson PA, Sasso RC, Riew KD. Comparison of adverse events between the Bryan artificial cervical disc and anterior cervical arthrodesis. *Spine.* 2008; 33:1305-12.

[2]   Apfelbaum RI, Kriskovich MD, Haller JR. On the incidence, cause, and prevention of recurrent laryngeal nerve palsies during anterior cervical spine surgery. *Spine.* 2000; 25: 2906-12.

[3]   Bazaz R, Lee MJ, Yoo JU. Incidence of dysphagia after anterior spine surgery: a prospective study. *Spine.* 2002; 27:2453-8.

[4]   BenDebba M, Heller J, Ducker TB, et al. Cervical spine outcomes questionnaire: its development and psychometric properties. *Spine.* 2002; 27:2116-23.

[5]   Carrau RL, Murry T: *Comprehensive Management of Swallowing Disorders.* San Diego, CA, Singular Publishing Group, 1999, pp11-29.

[6]   Chapman J, Hanson B, Dettori J, Norvell D, et al. *Spine outcomes measures and instruments.* New York, NY: Thieme; 2007:33-42.

[7]   Chen AY, Frankowski R, Bishop-Leone J, et al. The development and validation of a dyspagia-specific quality-of-life questionnaire for patients with head and neck cancer: the M.D. Anderson dysphagia inventory. *Arch. Otolaryngol. Head Neck Surg.* 2001; 127:870-6.

[8]   Chin KR, Eiszner JR, Adams SB, Role of plate thickness as a cause of dysphagia after anterior cervical fusion. *Spine* 2007; 32:2585-90.

[9]   Dailey AT, Hart D, Finn MA, et al. Anterior fixation of odontoid fractures in an elderly population. *World Spinal Column Journal.* 2010; 1:47-55.

[10]   Dettori JR, Norvell DC, Dekutoski M, et al. Methods for systematic reviews on patient safety during spine surgery. *Spine.* 2010; 35:s22-s27.

[11]   Dodds WJ, Logemann JA, Stewart ET. Radiologic assessment of abnormal oral and pharyngeal phases of swallowing. *AJR Am. J. Roentgenol.* 1990;154:965-74.

[12]   Edwards CC II, Karpitskaya Y, Cha C, et al: Accurate identification of adverse outcomes after cervical spine surgery. *J. Bone Joint. Surg. Am.* 2004; 86:251-256.

[13] Fogel GR, McDonnell MF. Surgical treatment of dysphagia after anterior cervical interbody fusion. *Spine J.* 2005; 5:140-4.

[14] Fountas KN, Kapsalaki EZ, Nikolakakos LG, et al. Anterior cervical discectomy and fusion associated complications. *Spine* 2007; 32:2310-7.

[15] Frempong-Boadu A, Houten JK, Osborn B, et al: Swallowing and speech dysfunction in patients undergoing anterior cervical discectomy and fusion: a prospective, objective preoperative and postoperative assessment. *J. Spinal Disord. Tech.* 2002; 15:362-368.

[16] Goyal RK. Disorders of the cricopharyngeus muscle. *Otolaryngol. Clin. North Am.* 1984;17:115-30.

[17] Haller JM, Iwanik M, Shen FH. Clinically relevant anatomy of high anterior cervical approach. *Spine.* 2011(feb 18).

[18] Kriskovich MD, Apfelbaum RI, Haller JR. Vocal fold paralysis after anterior cervical spine surgery: incidence, mechanism, and prevention of injury. *Laryngoscope.* 2000; 110:1467-73.

[19] Lee JY, Lim MR, Albert TJ: Dysphagia after anterior cervical spine surgery: pathophysiology, incidence, and prevention. http://www. csrs.org/web/outcomes/ clinsafetyoutcomespaper.pdf.

[20] Lee MJ, Bazaz R, Furey CG, Yoo J. Influence of anterior cervical plate design on dysphagia: a 2 year prospective longitudinal follow-up study. *J. Spinal Disord. Tech.* 2005; 18:406-9.

[21] Martin RE, Neary MA, Diamant NE. Dysphagia following anterior cervical spine surgery. *Dysphagia.* 1997; 12:2-10.

[22] Mummaneni PV, Burkus JK, Haid RW, et al. Clinical and radiographic analysis of cervical disc arthroplasty compared with allograft fusion: a randomized controlled clinical trial. *J. Neurosurg. Spine.* 2007; 6:198-209.

[23] Okubadejo GO, Hohl JB, Donaldson WF: *Dysphonia, dysphagia, and esophageal injuries after anterior cervical spine surgery. AAOS Instructional Course Lectures*, Vol 58, 2009.

[24] Palmer JB, Drennan JC Baba M, Evaluation and treatment of swallowing impairments. *Am. Fam. Physician* 2000; 61:2453-62.

[25] Pedram M, Castagnera L, Carat X, et al. Pharyngolaryngeal lesions in patients undergoing cervical spine surgery through the anterior approach: contribution of methylprednisolone. *Eur. Spine. J.* 2003; 12:84-90.

[26] Ratnaraj J, Todorov A, McHugh T, et al. Effects of decreasing endotracheal tube cuff pressures during neck retraction for anterior cervical spine surgery. *J. Neurosurg.* 2002:97(2 suppl):176-9.

[27] Riley, LH III, Skolasky RL, Albert TJ, Vaccaro AR, Heller JG. Dysphagia after anterior cervical decompression and fusion: prevalence and risk factors from a longitudinal cohort study. *Spine.* 2005; 30:2564-9.

[28] Riley LH, Vaccaro AR, Dettori JR, et al. Postoperative dysphagia in anterior cervical spine surgery. *Spine.* 2010; 95:576-85.

[29] Rhyne AL, Spector LR, Schmidt GL et al. Anatomic mapping and evaluation of the exophagus in relation to the cervical vertebral body. *Eur. Spine. J.* 2007: 16:1267-72.

[30] Segebarth B, Datta JC, Darden B. Incidence of dysphagia comparing cervical arthroplasty and ACDF. *SAS Journal.* 2010; 4:3-8.

[31] Smith-Hammond CA, New KC, Pietrobon R, et al. Prospective analysis of incidence and risk factors of dysphagia in spine surgery patients: comparison of anterior cervical, posterior cervical, and lumbar procedures. *Spine.* 2004: 29:1441-6.

[32] Smucker JD, Rhee JM, Singh K, Yoon ST, Heller JG. Increased swelling complications associated with off-label usage of rh-BMP-2 in the anterior cervical spine. *Spine.* 2006; 31:2813-9.

[33] Weisberg NK, Spengler DM, Netterville JL. Stretch-induced nerve injury as a cause of paralysis secondary to the anterior cervical approach. *Otolaryngol. Head Neck Surg.* 1997; 116:317-26.

[34] Yue WM, Brodner W, Highland TR. Persistent swallowing and voice problems after anterior cervical discectomy and fusion with allograft and plating: a 5-11 year follow-up study. *Eur. Spine. J.* 2005; 14:677-82.

In: Dysphagia   ISBN: 978-1-61942-104-2
Editors: B. S. Smith and M. Adams   © 2012 Nova Science Publishers, Inc.

Chapter VI

THE CONTRIBUTION OF DEGLUTITION SOUNDS FOR THE ASSESSMENT OF DYSPHAGIA, ASPIRATION AND PENETRATION: A LITERATURE REVIEW*

Christiane Borr
Department of Clinical Linguistics,
Faculty of Linguistics and Literary Studies,
Bielefeld Univ., Bielefeld, Germany

Abstract

The clinical swallow examination (CSE) is often the only tool given to speech and language therapists to identify patients with a high risk of aspiration, penetration and dysphagia. With the help of the CSE, the clinician is able to gauge the oral phase. However, it is difficult to assess the pharyngeal phase because it is impossible see what is happening. Several

*A version of this chapter also appears in *Educational Evaluation: 21st Century Issues and Challenges*, edited by María Oritiz and Claudia Rubio, published by Nova Science Publishers, Inc. It was submitted for appropriate modifications in an effort to encourage wider dissemination of research.

studies report poor sensitivity – that is, the ability to identify true aspirators, and poor specificity – the ability to classify true non-aspirators. Even experienced clinicians can identify aspiration with the assessment of clinical parameters in only 40–60% of the radiologically verified examples. This is why we would be grateful for rapid and reliable methods and procedures that boost the sensitivity and specificity of the clinical assessment. Many publications propose several methods – one of them cervical auscultation (CA). In this article I am reviewing about 40 years of experience with and research on the knowledge of CA. The focus will be on studies employing the methodical basis of CA, acoustic analysis, or imaging techniques. Finally, I will discuss the diagnostic contribution of CA to the assessment of swallowing disorders and delineate further research prospects.

1. Introduction

Dysphagia is a symptom of various diseases which increases morbidity as well as mortality. It is a risk factor for aspiration pneumonia, upper airway obstruction, malnutrition and dehydration [Mueller and Lorenz, 2005] and psychosocial effects [Ekberg et al., 2002].

The proportion of people who suffer from dysphagia aged 55+ is about 16–22% and for those aged 75+ about 45%. With stroke patients the proportion varies between 16 and 100%, for patients with amyotrophic lateral sclerosis it is given as 48–100%. Every second patient with Parkinson's disease also suffers from dysphagia. Stroke is the most common cause of neurogenous dysphagia [Mueller and Lorenz, 2005]. In Germany approximately 5 million people – that is about 7% of all citizens! – suffer from dysphagia [http://www.ernaehrungsmed.de/content/view/23/213 (accessed January 16, 2006)]. Accordingly, it is estimated that circa 13–14% of the patients who are in acute clinics and up to 50% of the residents of nursing homes suffer from oral intake disabilities. About 50% of the survivors of a stroke event that are treated in a stroke unit are affected by dysphagia as a consequence of paralysis. In the USA the situation is similar [Kaplan et al., 2002, Marik and Kaplan, 2003]. The incidence clearly depends on age and reaches its peak between 60 and 75 years. Only one in a thousand senior adults living at home suffer from aspiration pneumonia every year, as opposed to 33 in a thousand of nursing home patients [Kaplan et al., 2002]. The health economic effect of the increasing life expectancy is quite impressive, as exemplified by community aquired pneumonia: In the USA the annual costs for the treatment of ambulant aquired pneumonia are estimated at 4.4 billion US Dollars [Marrie, 2000]. In this context it has to be stressed that pneumonia is just one of the complications mentioned earlier! If dysphagia is recognized in time, these complications and their unwelcome impact on the patient can be avoided.

All-important in dysphagia are deglutition disorder that results in aspiration of oropharyngeal or gastral residues into the lower respiratory tract. Aspiration is generally an underestimated cause of community-acquired pneumonia. Aspiration pneumonia is caused by aspiration, i.e. the penetration of meals and drinks into the lower respiratory tract. If after the development of a deglutition paralysis even the spontaneous swallowing of saliva is diminished, a densification of the pathogenic germs of the natural oral flora may occur as quickly as within three to four hours after the stroke incident [Hammond et al., 2005]. As soon as this "pathogenic saliva" is swallowed and invades the lungs a highly aggressive pneumonia may be induced in a little short time [Hammond et al., 2005]. There is evidence that early recognized dysphagia in survivors of an acute stroke has a favourable impact not only on the outcome of the treatment with regard to pneumonia, mortality, and length of hospital stay, but also on the expense of the whole in-patient treatment [Martino et al., 2000].

The recognition and the therapy of a particular type of dysphagia is based on the complete assessment of the swallow functions. This is a complex process that requires the specialised skills of a qualified speech and language therapist. Systemic review articles by [Doggett et al., 2002] and [Martino et al., 2000] first recommend to apply fast and simple screening methods in order to identify those patients with high risk of aspiration, penetration and dysphagia. More intensive assessment of the swallow functions should be carried out later. The timely and exact identification of dysphagia with the help of screening assessments allows an early initiation of prophylactic actions and adequate care directly after the stroke event. In addition, it shortens reconvalescence of the patient from the consequences of the stroke and reduces the rehabilitation costs. Several sources give evidence that a timely dysphagia screening in acute stroke survivors accounts for a significant relative risk reduction of pneumonia of more than 80%, a significant relative risk reduction for mortality of 70%, a reduction of PEG insertion, and a reduction of the whole health care costs[Hammond et al., 2005]. Only interdisciplinary cooperation and a differentiated as well as targeted diagnosis can deal with the broad variety of symptoms of dysphagia. The question, however, is with which methods or procedures can assist in diagnosing patients that suffer from the multifactory symtomatic complex called dysphagia in such a way that they can be safely assigned into a specific pathogenous group. This method also has to show a sensible cost-benefit ratio. If the suspicion of an incidence of dysphagia arises the *American Speech Language and Hearing Association* (ASHA) generally advises to use a clinical examination besides an instrumental diagnosis to assess the swallow function and the risk of pneumonia caused by aspiration (ASHA, 2000). The diagnostic procedures used should follow (at least) the following four guidelines. The procedures should complement each other, they should form an integral part of the steps in clinical treatment, a standardized testing should be guaranteed (if possible), and the diagnostic assessment tools should determine the treatment techniques and their evaluation. A useful diagnostic procedure has to be reliable (i.e. the procedure yields equal results on repeated trials) as well as valid (this means in the present case that the procedure detects dysphagia if and only if it is actually there). A number of methods proposed to describe dysphagia, especially aspiration, are neither reliable nor valid e.g., the 3-oz water swallow test [DePippo et al., 1992] or the repetitive saliva swallowing test (RSST)[Oguchi et al., 2000]. Pulse oximetry has also been proposed as a method of identifying the aspiration risk at the bedside [Perry and Love, 2001, Lim et al., 2001, Sherman et al., 1999]. However, several studies comparing the results of pulse oximetry with the established imaging techniques found evidence that there is no strict correlation between arterial oxygen saturation and the occurrence of aspiration (regarding functional fiberoptic endoscopic evaluation of swallowing (fFEES) see [Colodny, 2000, Leder, 2000]; regarding videofluoroscopy (VFES) cf. [Sellars et al., 1998]). Current publications give a number of inconsistent recommendations – compare the overview given in [Mathers-Schmidt and Kurlinski, 2003]. Actually, only a few of these methods have been proven to fulfill the desired criteria, (i.e. reliability, validity and objectivity). To name one: the water swallow test by Daniels et al. [Daniels et al., 1997] for acute stroke patients. In the apparative diagnosis, on the other hand, two complementary methods are established on equals: VFES, the so called gold standard [Scott et al., 1998], and fFEES [Langmore88, Aviv]. Both methods have their own advantages and disadvantages in view of the evaluation of relevant parameters such as risk of aspiration and penetration or the assessment of the bolus transport time. Furthermore, both methods share two problems with all other procedures: First, there is no standard for quantifying measuring values. Second, none of them complies with the conditions of reliability and validity, see [Stoeckli et al., 2003] in regard to VFES and [Colodny, 2000] in regard to fFEES. In addition, both methods have some further disadvantages in that they could not be employed with every patient and they are not available in most ordinary hospitals. One example is VFES, it is expensive, unsuitable as a bedside screening and linked to radiation [Stroud et al., 2002]. In some clinical institutions, other methods are also in use for the assessment of swallowing and for swallowing research, e.g., ultrasonics [Böhme, 1990], scintigraphy, and manometry. All these methods require costly equipment and highly trained stuff to interpret their outcomes. In recent years an alternative has been sought. An objective apparative diagnosis procedure for assessing the fundamental swallow functions. One method especially has been given some attention by researchers: *cervical auscultation* [Stroud et al., 2002, Leslie et al., 2004, Takahashi et al., 1994a]. Cervical auscultation (CA) is a method of listening to the sounds of swallowing and swallow-related respiration between the throat and the larynx. It is conducted during the pharyngeal phase with an amplifying instrument in order to detect patients with a high aspiration and penetration risk. Such instruments are, for example, stethoscopes or microphones. They are placed at the lateral aspect above the cricoid cartilage in front of the sternocleidomastoid muscle and the large blood vessels. CA is common in the Anglo-American countries and in European countries, particularly in Germany where it is considered an additional diagnostic tool. Generally it is recognized as a limited but popular method for aspiration detection and dysphagia assessment in long-term care, see, e.g., [Zenner et al., 1995, Cichero and Murdoch, 2002a, Stroud et al., 2002].

2.   Historical Outline

Auscultation already has a bit of experience under its belt. Since the invention of the stethoscope by R. T. H. Laennec (presumably in the year 1816) the method has frequently been used for the diagnosis of heart and pulmonary diseases. The auscultation of noises associated with swallowing has a long tradition. At the beginning of the twentieth century A. F. Hertz analysed the sounds that are caused by the passage of bites into the food channel (Hertz, 1907). In the case of liquids being swallowed, he observed that the sounds are brief and sharp and coincide with the contraction of the *M. mylohyoideus* as well as with the elevation of the larynx.

About forty years ago CA was the subject of experimental research by physicians [Lear et al., 1965, Logan et al., 1967, Mackowiak et al., 1967] – with simple means, from today's point of view; The sounds which accompany the physiological actions of coughing, sipping, breathing and vocalising were recorded with the help of a stethoscope and subseqently represented as a spectrum. The physicians found a characteristic and distinctive pattern for each of the various actions. The pattern of the swallow sounds in particular exhibited changes related to the quantity and the consistency of the bolus.

The first study from the area of speech and language pathology was given to us by Sandra Hamlet and her colleagues in the 90's. Since that time studies on CA have been published regularly. The studies can be divided into three categories: (1) studies with methodical and instrumental considerations [Hamlet et al., 1992, Takahashi et al., 1994a] – which place is the best to listen to the sounds and which instrument is suitable?; (2) evaluation studies in connection with imaging techniques like VFES or fFEES [Hamlet et al., 1992, Vice and Bosma, 1995, Zenner et al., 1995, Stroud et al., 2002, Leslie et al., 2004]; and (3) studies focusing on acoustic analysis [Youmans and Stierwalt, 2005, Cichero and Murdoch, 2002a, Cichero and Murdoch, 2003, Kley and Biniek, 2005, Moriniére et al., 2006].

3.   Neuroanatomical Basics

Swallowing is an act that is controlled by several physiological and motor processes. This section gives a rough introduction to the neuroanatomical struc-

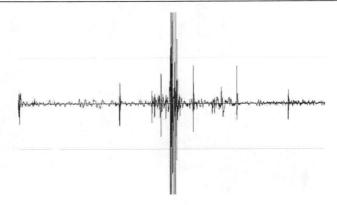

Figure 1. Waveform of the deglutition sound of a healthy, young man.

tures underlying a swallowing act. They will be approached from their "output", that is, the perceivable sounds. Some figures of waveforms of actual deglutitions serve to illustrate the discussion. A waveform is the visual representation of a sound's pressure over time. The first figure (Figure 1) shows a healthy degluti- tion of a 28 year-old man. The second figure (Figure 2) is the waveform of a 84 year-old woman suffering from cerebral infarction and the third one (Figure 3) is taken from the swallow sound of a 75 year-old man with Parkinson's disease.

Until today, there is no consensus on which physiologic event causes which sound. Deglutition does have an acoustic pattern – but researchers disagree about the single components of the acoustic pattern. There is some indication that the acoustic pattern of the dysphagics is very different from the healthy ones, as we can see in Figures 1 to 3.

Acoustic Characteristics

As with the voice, the sounds from swallowing also seem to be singu- lar to each individual. There is, nevertheless, a set of characteristic features which are typical for a healthy swallow sound. The healthy swallow sounds are very short and crisp [Cichero, 2006]. Measurements of the duration of deg- lutition resulted in an average of 0.4 seconds [Cichero and Murdoch, 2002b] until 0.5 seconds [Youmans and Stierwalt, 2005], a stable intensity of 43 dB [Cichero and Murdoch, 2002b] to 61 dB [Youmans and Stierwalt, 2005] and an

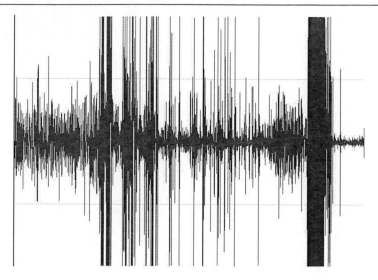

Figure 2. Waveform of the deglutition sound of of a elderly woman suffering from cerebral infarction.

Table 1. The swallowing sound duration as a function on the swallowers' ages, taken from [Cichero and Murdoch, 2002a]

1 year	18–35 years	36–59 years	60+ years
0.12 s [Willett, 2002]	0.37 s	0.48 s	0.52 s

average frequency of 2200 Hz [Cichero and Murdoch, 2002b] up to 2300 Hz [Youmans and Stierwalt, 2005]. To compare: identical values develop with the phonation of /i:/, e.g., the sound of the letter *y* at the end of the name *Andy*. The configuration of the tongue and of the oral structures with formation of the vowel corresponds to the starting position when swallowing. The two clicks are even audible for the non-professionals [Borr et al., 2007]. However, swallowed might be so fast that both sounds blur and sound like just a single acoustic event. Swallow sounds depend on physiological conditions that are subject to change during aging (see Table [Cichero, 2006]) and depend on what is swallowed, and on the quantity swallowed.

The   studies   of   [Cichero and Murdoch, 2002b]   and

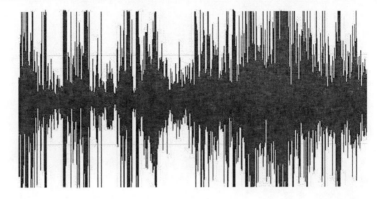

Figure 3. Waveform of the deglutition sound of a man suffering from Parkinson's disease

[Youmans and Stierwalt, 2005] revealed that the duration of the swallowing sound increases significantly with age, but it would probably require a lot of training and experience to notice these differences in the patient. Some evidence that deglutition becomes shorter if the volume of the bolus increases is also reported [Cichero and Murdoch, 2003]. However, there is disagreement among researchers about *how* the consistency of the bolus influences the swallowing sound duration and the frequency.

[Cichero and Murdoch, 2002a] maintain that the deglutition sound is shorter and less frequent if the liquid swallowed was of thicker consistency. However, Youmans and Stierwalt [Youmans and Stierwalt, 2005] could not confirm that the consistency of the bolus affected duration and frequency of the deglutition parameters. Some studies analysed the acoustic characteristics of the swallow sounds of dysphagics suffering from dysphagia of different severity. Both common and different features of aspirators/penetrators with dysphagia and dysphagics without aspiration (severe vs. mild dysphagia) were looked for, also features which might help to differentiate between dysphagic and healthy subjects. Both groups of dysphagia patients have two characteristics in common as compared to the healthy participants, namely a longer duration of deglutition (dysphagics: 0.92 s and aspirators: 0.6 s healthy: 0.4) and more highly frequent swallow sound in direction [Cichero and Murdoch, 2002a]. A study by [Borr et al., 2007] points into a similar direction.

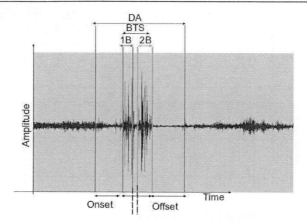

Figure 4. Schematic despiction of a deglutition waveform [Borr et al., 2007]. Interburst is the nearly silent section between the bursts. The phase in which respiration is interrupted is called deglutition apnea (DA). A swallow's main events are the two bursts that are presumably correlated with the transport of the bolus through the pharynx. The periods of time from initiation of DA to the leading edge of the first burst and from the trailing edge of the second burst to the end of DA are called onset and offset, respectively.

Assuming that CA is indeed a successful procedure, the relevant information that shows whether a swallow is dysphagic or not should be divulged by the swallowing sound itself. To put it another way: The swallow sound exhibits objectively audible characteristics which permit a distinction between pathological and healthy swallows. The study of [Borr et al., 2007] searches for objective acoustic characteristics in the temporal structure of the swallow sounds. Swallowing sounds of fourteen dysphagic patients, 25 of younger healthy subjects and 25 of older healthy subjects were annotated following the pattern suggested by [McKaig, 2002] (see Figure 4).

A quantitative comparison of this "swallow morphology" between the groups resulted in only few significant differences – too few for a reliable diagnosis. However, it has recently been reported that SLTs are, in principle, able to successfully use CA – see for example the reliability, sensitivity and specificity values given in [Leslie et al., 2004] and [Stroud et al., 2002]. In a second part of the same study, experienced CA experts were asked to classify swallow sounds and enter their observations into questionnaires [Borr et al., 2007]. The experts classified 33 swallow sounds to decide whether the sound came from a dysphagic, a young healthy subject, or an older one. In this second part the sensitivity and specificity of the expert classification were determined – reliability being measured as the degree of agreement between the ratings (inter-rater agreement). The results for objective acoutic characteristics (see above) imply that it is improbable that the experts rely on the swallow sounds alone. Consequently, all raters were asked on which criteria they based their classifications. The study as a whole examines the following questions:

- Are there any objective acoustic properties that distinguish between dysphagic and nondysphagic deglutitions?

- Are there any acoustic properties that distinguish bewcen older and younger subjects' deglutitions?

- To what extent do CA experts agree in classifying swallowing sounds?

- Do the raters (experts and the layperson) classify swallowing sounds correctly?

- Does acquaintance with CA improve classifications?

- On which parameters do raters base their classifications?

The following section describes the methodical structure of the study.

A data collection with the recordings of swallow sounds of different groups of swallowers were arranged for the CA analysis, namely a dysphagic group and two healthy control groups of different ages.

The test data consists of the swallowing sounds of fourteen dysphagic patients, ten females and four males. The dysphagic participants were in average 71.3 years (range: 44 to 89 years).

The subjects had neurogenic dysphagia due to a cerebrovascular primary disease. Dysphagia resulted from an anemic infarct or a hemorrhage. The onset of the event was no longer than three months ago. All patients showed clinical signs of a dysphagia and had an aspiration risk. Clinical assessment of the patients was conducted using VFSS. In all patients severe dysphagia with penetration and aspiration was diagnosed. The time between swallow recording and image-giving assessment was, at most, one week. The results of the videofluoroscopic examination were recorded on hospital-internal non-standardized data sheets. If the findings are to be translated into the standardized penetration and aspiration scale – similiar to the one [Rosenbek et al., 1996] introduced – the patients have to be classified at least at level 6. Subjects with progressive neurogenic diseases and patients with chronic dysphagia were excluded.

The test data of the younger subjects are 25 swallowing sounds that were randomly selected from the author's corpus of 250 swallow recordings. The younger subjects did not have a history of neurological problems. The younger volunteers (students and staff of the University) were tested at the University of Bielefeld. The analysed data contain the swallow recordings of eleven women and fourteen men. The mean age of the younger subject was 30.9 years (range: 25 to 44 years).

The swallow recordings of 25 older subjects (13 females and 12 males) without previous neurological and dysphagic problems constitute the older control group. The age of the older participants was in average 76.2 years (range: 60 to 97 years). The older volunteers were recruited among the patients of a local family doctor. Due to ethical and financial reasons no imaging was performed. The suitability of the volunteers for the participation in the study was exclusively based on their medical documents.

3.1.   Procedure and Devices

Each swallow of all subjects was recorded in a controlled and specified way.   In the first place, the larynx was located and the so-called four-finger method, i.e., the palpation of the laryngeal elevation [Perlman and Schulze-Delrieu, 1997] was applied.   The four-finger method helps to receive a "haptic impression" of the laryngeal movements in order to locate the most suitable place for the stethoscope. This procedure helps to build confidence between therapist and patient. The study leader placed the stethoscope (Welch Allyn Meditron) at the lateral aspect over the cricoid cartilage [Takahashi et al., 1994a] in front of the sternocleidomastoid muscle and the large neck vessels. The patients were handed three portions of 10 ml tab water each. The swallows were recorded with an Audiorecorder (a Windows XP tool) on a commercial Notebook (Toshiba 1900 Satellite). The mono line-in had a resolution of 16 bits and a scanning rate of 44.1 kHz. The frequency covered a range from 20 Hz to 20 kHz. The high-pass filter in the stethoscope was activated during the recordings. The subjects were told to swallow in a normal fashion to approximate their "natural" drinking behaviour.

4. Parameter Structuring

The sound files were displayed as spectrum and annotated using the software program Soundforge 6.0. A schematic representation of a prototypical waveform is given in Figure 4. The term 'spectrum' is used synonymously with the term 'waveform' [Clark and Yallop, 1995]. A waveform is the visual representation of acoustic pressure over time with the intensity of the pressure in decibel on the y-axis and the time in milliseconds on the x axis. Each physiological event correlates with an acoustic signal [McKaig, 2002], and some caution would have to be exercised (see above). According to [McKaig, 2002] the pharyngeal phase divides into five sections, see Figure 4. Tidal breathing, which is present before the release of the swallow reflex, is the first section. The following breath interruption happens when the configuration of the pharynx changes from the air channel into the swallow channel. The phase of the deglutition apnea continues over the whole pharyngeal phase. The first burst is to be heard as blasting noise. It probably correlates with the penetration of the bolus into the hypopharynx [McKaig, 2002].The second burst follows after a short interval, which marks the passage of the bolus through the hypopharynx. The two bursts represent the third and fourth section in the waveform.

In the following quiet stripping wave (the so-called offset time, the fifth section), the hypopharynx is being emptied. The bolus is pushed towards the esophagus – its opening is a complex phenomenon itself [Mu and Sanders, 1998]. During the last phase of the opening procedure the upper esophagus sphincter is closed and a continuous muscle tonus is re-established. If the nasopharynx is closed again, the glottis opens, tidal breathing sets again, and the pharyngeal phase terminates.

When the clinicians auscultate the swallow sounds, qualitative judgements are made about what is heard. The characteristic swishing doubleclick (the two bursts) of the bolus passing through the pharynx and into the esophagus is judged for normalcy, based on the crispness of the sound. A reliable definition is not yet given in physical terms, but generally it is characterized as a short,

Table 2. The parameters for structuring deglutition waveforms, taken from [Borr et al., 2007]

Parameters	Abbrev.	Description
Onset time	ON	Period of time from initiation of deglutition apnea to leading edge of first burst
Deglutition Apnea	DA	Duration of time from initiation to the end of deglutition apnea
First Burst	1B	Duration of initial burst
Second Burst	2B	Duration of second burst
Bolus transport signal	BTS	Duration of time from leading edge of first burst to trailing edge of second burst
Offset time	OFF	Period of time from trailing edge of second burst to end of deglutition apnea
Deglutition	D	Number of gulps used to gulp down the bolus

high-frequent cracking [Hamlet et al., 1994].

The cardinal points for the annotation were determined as following [McKaig, 2002] (compare Figure 4). They consist of marking the beginning and the end of the deglutition apnea, and the time spans of the first and the second burst. The intervals of the other relevant sections of the pharyngeal phase were calculated from those four points (see Table 2) which were annotated independently by two raters. The calculation of Cronbach's alpha [Cronbach, 1951] on both annotations resulted in values above 0.9 for all seven parameters and can, therefore, be interpreted as consistently following the line of thought in Langer [Langer, 2003].

5. Results

Comparing the parameters annotated on the deglutition sounds of the younger and the older groups, [Borr et al., 2007] find two relevant differences: First, durations of the deglutition apnea differs significantly ($p = 0.047$) and second, the onset time ($p = 0.1$) shows a difference in direction. Both relevant values are higher in the older group than in the younger one.

Between the younger and the dysphagic group the duration of the deglutition apnea ($p = 0.07$) and the onset time ($p = 0.03$) show relevant differences,

Table 3. Comparison of the parameters for all groups with X for significant and Y for a tendency

Parameter	younger vs older	younger vs dysphagic	older vs dysphagic
DA	X	Y	–
ON	X	Y	–
1B	–	–	X
D	–	X	X

too. One parameter which differentiates significantly whether the swallow stems from a young or dysphagic participant is the parameter number of gulps ($p = 0.001$). Dysphagics often need more than one gulp to swallow the bolus. There are two parameters that distinguish swallowing sounds of the older from the dysphagic group: first and above all, the duration of the first burst ($p = 0.1$), and second, multiple gulps ($p = 0.00$). Dysphagic patients need more than one gulp to swallow the bolus and they show a slightly shorter first burst. The results are summarised in Table 3.[1]

So far the swallow sounds were represented as isolated events that take place in the pharyngeal phase at the beginning of the esophageal phase (and presented accordingly in relevant studies). Today, the events are regarded as being contextualised with all other swallow phases. There are further important audible features from the pre-oral and the oral phase, not to forget breath and swallow coordination. Before healthies start to swallow one can hear a series of sounds that are related to breathing, masticating, tongue movements, bolus preparation and/or to the admission of liquid and food into the oral cavity.

In the dysphagic patients, on the other hand, we would expect wheezing and modified breathings, e.g., stridor and wet sounds of breathing and streaming sounds of the bolus in the dysphagic patient [Cichero, 2006].The oropharyngeal transit times (i.e., the intervals between the bolus starting to enter the oral cavity to the instant the swallow sound can be heard) are longer in the dysphagic and aspirate patient than in the healthy ones [Cichero, 2006].

---

[1]The mean values of the relevant seven parameters for the three groups are represented as Table 2 in [Borr et al., 2007]. The factor analysis (one-factorial ANOVA) calculated was followed by *post hoc* Scheffé tests for each parameter. The statistic results are represented in Table 3 in [Borr et al., 2007].

After swallow the sound of the glottal release (described above) can be heard in the healthy subjects. This sound is reported by [Cichero and Murdoch, 2003] to have a duration of 0.2 seconds.

With 38 dB it is softer than the clicks [Cichero and Murdoch, 2003]. The clinician hears a short air blast directly after the swallow, before the tidal breathing starts again. With dysphagics this sound is missing either completely or is very quiet and short. The glottal release sound in the group of the aspirators is often extremely loud (almost explosive). Both in aspirators (0.53 seconds) and in dysphagics (0.74 seconds) [Cichero and Murdoch, 2003] were able to measure a clearly longer glottal release sound compared to the healthy group. If that sound is missing, the authors assume a longer closure of the respiratory tract. The subjects of the healthy group resume tidal breathing immediately after the glottal release sound.

With patients who are dysphagics and aspirators most sounds are expected to accompany coughs, harrumph, bubbling, gurgling, wet breathing, stridor or gasps, or to arise out of the respiration rate after the deglutition. The duration of the entire deglutition is a useful measure for hints on swallow safeness and the efficiency of the swallow. For the healthy group the swallow sound duration, measured by affecting the bolus of the lip up to the reinsertion of the tidal breathing, is indicated with 2.47 seconds [Cichero, 2006]. In dysphagics, however, it lasts much longer (9.94 seconds). Aspirators in general need more time for swallowing (total period: 12.23 seconds), and in particular it takes them longer to find back to normal tidal breathing.

6.   Equipment for Recording

One essential for hearing swallow sounds is an appropriate instrument. Today, stethoscopes and microphones are available, and also accelerometers, which were developed to record the vibrations of swallowing and breathing. In the day-to-day business of clinics, stethoscopes are used most, while accelerometers are more often employed for research purposes. Data acquisition by microphone, electronic stethoscope, and accelerometer can be fed directly into the computer and subsequently be visualised via computer digitization functions. The data are available for direct evaluation. The audio channel of a video recorder (e.g., during the VFES) and the audio channel of a Handicam camera can also both be used for data input with microphones and accelerometers. [Hamlet et al., 1994] examined altogether six of the commercial stethoscopes and compared their acoustic characteristics. In detail, they dealt with the following questions:

1. How well does the frequency response of the stethoscope reflect the frequency which actually occurs in the swallow sound?

2. Are there significant differences in the frequency responses of the stethoscopes?

3. Which stethoscope is suited best for the requirements of CA?

The assessment of the stethoscopes took place in accordance with six criteria on an ordinal assessment scale of the frequency response characteristics of the respective instrument. In the low frequency range a reinforcement of very low frequencies and a good regularity of lower to middle frequencies are necessary. Accordingly, the stethoscopes had to meet the following criteria :

1. reinforcement of noises below 100 Hz,

2. absorption <10 dB in the range of 100–700 Hz with a variability of 0–10 dB,

3. absorption <15 dB in the range of 100–700 Hz with a variability of 5–15 dB.

In the higher frequency range, a relative lack of absorption and a good regularity of frequency response within the middle frequencies are necessary, so the stethoscopes had to comply with the following:

1. absorption <30 dB in the range of 1800–3000 Hz,

2. absorptoin <20 dB in the range of 1000–1800 Hz,

3. absorption <15 dB in the range of 100–700 Hz with a variability of 5–15 dB.

The six criteria mentioned above are currently only met by two stetho-scopes, namely *Littman Cardiology II* and *Hewlett Packard Rappaport Sprague* (medium Bell, small diaphragm). [Hamlet et al., 1994] noticed in conclusion that clinicians arrive at assessments based on what they hear. The characteristic, switching double-click that happens if the bolus arrives at the pharynx and then enters into the esophagus, is, at least in healthy persons' swallows, the basis for the "crispness" of the noise. This feature can be picked up for classification or diagnosis. In comparison with accelerometers and microphones the frequency rendering of all kinds of stethoscopes is not well suited for intermediaries of high frequencies. Even the favourites listed above transfer high frequencies in a weakened fashion. Stethoscopes are suitable rather for the transmission of extremely low frequencies. [Hamlet et al., 1994] refer to the fact that the hu-man hearing is most sensitive for the sounds between 2000–3000 Hz, the spec-trum in which also the main sound energy of swallowing is situated. Therefore [Hamlet et al., 1994] advises the use of a filter or a funnel for optimal rendering of swallow sound.

6.1. Microphones and Accelerometers

The use of miniature accelerometers or different microphone systems offers further possibilities for the assessment of swallow sounds by auscultation or transduction from the body suface[Hamlet et al., 1992]. It is possible to save the acoustic signal for subsequent analysis, the signal can be played back directly over headphones or loudspeakers for the purpose of immediate use, and the signal can even be used as a biofeedback signal for therapeutic uses.

6.1.1. Accelerometer

An accelerometer is an acceleration adaptor. It measures the vibration of a surface and is sensitive to a far range of frequencies. If a very small accelera-tion adaptor is attached to the neck with a double tape,, the sensor transforms the vibration induced by the swallow sounds on the skin surface into electric-ity [McKaig, 2002]. This procedure is optimal if the sensor directly rests on a firm structure, for example the larynx. [Smith et al., 2000] underline that the ac-celerometer is to be preferred over other techniques since it supresses surround-ing noise more effectively and is only activated from the surface vibrations on the skin. In addition, an accelerometer provides regular acoustic signals. The disadvantages of accelerometers are to be seen in their very difficult handling and high costs. To be added are the difficult adjustment of the sensor at the skin and the fact that the best sensor placement is not yet found and in most cases a reinforcement of the signal is necessary. In clinical studies cervical auscultation with the use of an accelerometer for the recording of the swallowing sounds yielded moderate agreement with videofluoroscopy in detecting patients with a risk of aspiration [Reddy et al., 1994]. The amplitude of the accelerometer signal is linked to the extent of the cranio-ventral movement of the larynx [Reddy et al., 2000].

6.1.2. Contact Microphone

A microphone makes the direct recording of acoustic signals on the skin surface possible, without further materials or media between the receivers and the skin surface. For data recording a contact microphone is most suitable because of its good frequency response even with lower frequencies. A great disadvantage is the relatively high weight due to which a contact microphone is difficult to attach.

7. Optimal Position for Auscultation

Several opinions exist as to the positioning of the stethoscope head or the microphone/accelerometer for best results – in any case, somewhere in the laryngo-pharyngeal area. A problematic area – it is not exactly large and consistently disturbed by permanent acoustic activity. A considerable part of the acoustic activity is due to flow sounds of liquids and gases. In close neighbourhood to the suitable laryngopharyngeal area lie not only the carotids, the lymphatics and *V. jugularis interna*, which produce arterial and venous container sounds, but also the spinal fluid. In addition, air interchange is carried out there. The ensemble of these activities often causes disturbing noises for the CA. "Acousticians characterize such a relationship by the so-called signal-to-noise ratio" [McKaig, 2000]. That means, something simplified, if existing interferences are decreased, it is easier to recognize the acoustic signal. This concept can be illustrated by the example of listening to the radio while driving a car: The closer one comes to the radio station, the less white noise is to be heard. Due to anatomical characteristics, many sounds compete with the swallow sounds. Therefore, it is essential to carefully place the receiver where a good signal-to-noise ratio can be obtained. [Takahashi et al., 1994a] examined 24 suitable placements on the lateral aspect on the neck of 14 healthy adults in order to identify the best place for the recording of swallow sounds. Figure 5 shows the appropriate locality.

Takahashi and his coworkers told the subjects to drink 5 ml liquid with one gulp three times. The swallow sounds were recorded with a TEAC 501 accelerometer, which was connected to a TEAC SA-16 amplifier with a DSP sonagraph Kay 5500. They arrived at the following results:

1. The locality labelled 11 in Figure 5 in the *Trigonum submandibulare*, laterally in a middle line between sign and ring cartilages before *M. sternocleidomastoideus*, and the carotid artery, shows the strongest amplitude and the smallest standard deviation in the signal-to-noise ratio. Therefore, Takahashi and his team consider this place best for applying a CA.

2. The localization places 4 (center of the ring cartilage) and 5 (center between four and six) are regarded as suitable as well, due to their good values in the signal-to-noise ratio.

The authors point out that for the assessment of respiration or swallow sounds with infants and babies further localization places could be applicable. McKaig [McKaig, 2002] favours a stethoscope placement laterally between the larynx and behind the trachea anterior to a carotid side. With regard to further research of [Takahashi et al., 1994b] this placement dependens on factors like the size of the instrument and the relative size of the patient's neck. [Cichero and Murdoch, 2002b] arrive at similar results as Takahashi and his colleagues. They found the middle placement on the trachea directly under the cricoid cartilage to be most suitable. In clinical practice the localisation of auscultation can vary from patient to patient. In some cases, the relevant sounds are heard best if the amplifying instrument is placed below the cricoid cartilage, in other cases a lateral placement for a clear sound is preferrable. [Cichero, 2006] confirms that the best location for auscultation is found if the tidal respiration can be differentiated clearly with a placement below the cricoid cartilage, whether in middle position or laterally.

8.   Annotation Tools

Each swallowing sound recording was saved in an uncompressed and computer-readable audio format (.wav files). After that, the analysis with a special program followed. The market provides various software programs for analysis, for example the audioprograms Soundforge or Audacity. [Morinière et al., 2007] used Cool Edit Pro software (Syntrillium Software Corporation, Phoenix, AZ, USA) for the analysis. The program should come with at least two features: First, it should be able to display the soundfiles as waveforms. Second, it should offer annotation facilities in order to mark the cardinal points. Other convenient features are, of course, desirable, like navigation and zooming facilities, amongst others.

To come back to an example already introduced above: In [Borr et al., 2007] the cardinal points were annotated independently by two raters with using a common strategy that relies on identifying the visual landmarks postulated by [McKaig, 2002]. This approach was adjusted after an exploratory annotation session. With this strategy, Cronbach's alpha [Cronbach, 1951] was above 0.9 for all parameters and that can be interpreted as consistent following the argument in [Langer, 2003].

Wishful would like to replace human annotations with machine based procedures (so called automatic recognition). Annotation is currently a manual process that combines two grave disadvantages. First, the procedure depends on the examiner' experience, i.e. subjective skills. Second, it is time-consuming.

It would be a great improvement to have an automated, reliable, objective and fast tool for annotation. It should be able to make decisions like trained SLTs, physicians or technicians.

Several sources propose several machine based procedures[Lazareck and Moussavi, 2004,   Lazareck and Ramanna, 2004, Lazareck and Moussavi, 2008] and[Lee et al., 2006].   The smart algorithm by[Lazareck and Moussavi, 2008]might be a promising candidate.

Three key signal features were extracted from the swallow signal to allow the classification process: The autoregressive (AR) coefficients, root-mean-square (RMS) values of the time signal, and the average power of the signal (P_{ave}) within a frequency band. However, [Lazareck and Moussavi, 2008] produced the classification sequences for the swallowing sounds of only six healthy subjects. They conducted two trials to investigate the separation into breath and swallow classes on the one side and in "click" and "non-click" classes on the other side. For the purpose of that research, initial and final clicks were considered as a single entity.

The reason of the selection of three sound signal features was that the time domain signal noticeably separates between sections, i.e., swallowing segments are, due to the clicks, much louder and, therefore, of a larger amplitude than segments while breathing. Besides, the breath segments are consistent in the frequency domain and the swallow segments are not. The authors compared the results with known values that were acquired by visual and auditory means. RMS in combination with the "smart" code yield an error rate of 21.55 % on average[Lazareck and Moussavi, 2008].

But though all the swallowing click sounds were classified correctly, some segments within the swallow sections and some segments in forceful expiration sections were not. Special difficulties are presented by sounds that were neither produced while breathing nor while swallowing, e.g. sounds that occur due to tongue movements [Lazareck and Moussavi, 2008]. The results of the study point into the right direction. Therefore, future studies aiming at a development of an automated program for the detection of swallowing sounds should involve a large-scale empirical study with subjects of various ages, because of age-related changes of the anatomical basis of a swallow.

Moreover, future work should include varying bolus textures, because swallowing sounds depend on the material being swallowed. One application goal is to create a program-user interface that assists in the process of decision making on classifying a swallowing sound as healthy or pathologic, and include the test of variations of the smart algorithm code to develop a robust algorithm cf. [Lazareck and Moussavi, 2008].

9.   Advantages and Disadvantages

CA offers a set of advantages. The method stands out since it is non-invasive and simple to handle. It also imposes low physical demand on the patient, which makes it suitable for severely diseased patients and even for toddlers. It is easily accepted by the patient, as for example, no disturbing tube needs to be inserted into the nose. The procedure is applicable at the bedside, if the patient can swallow at least saliva and small amounts of liquid. Using CA the patient can swallow a real bolus without the use of a contrast medium. CA can be applied as long as the SLT thinks it is necessary, because there is no radiation exposure. CA is flexible since it is not tied to a special place and can be taken to the patient. Finally it is repeatable, inexpensive and with proper training easy to use. Therefore CA is suitable for frequent use in hospitals and for therapy evaluation. For non-specialised hospitals and for ambulatory after-care CA can also be of great use. Compared to other procedures mentioned above CA is economical due to a minimum of personnel required and low initial costs for the material. With the help of CA the experienced clinician is able to judge the coordination between breathing and swallowing at the bedside.

Despite the large list of advantages of CA and despite the fact that it is a well-known method – due to being mentioned in the ASHA guidelines[ASHA, 2000] and other prominent publications – it is used only in isolated specialized clinics. The reason may be that clinicians need training and experience for a successful application. The user should also have good audition [Cichero, 2006]. In a study of [Richardson and Moody, 2000] the authors could prove that clinicians who play a musical instrument obtain higher classification successes than those who only received an audio teaching. Besides, still another open research question is to what extent CA fulfills the conditions of reliability and validity. When considered against videofluoroscopy, bedside assessment with stand-alone, CA yields limited accuracy in identification of aspirations [Zenner et al., 1995] and dysfunctions of swallowing [Leslie et al., 2004].

The sensitivity of CA for the identification of aspiration is indicated in several sources as 84%–87% [Zenner et al., 1995, Eicher et al., 1994]. Its specificity takes values between 56% [Zenner et al., 1995] and 78% [Eicher et al., 1994]. In a comparative study of [Eicher et al., 1994], the CA used as a supplement in the clinical diagnostics can identify occurrences of aspiration more accurately than CA stand alone. The imaging technique VFES is still gold standard for clinical examinations. Table 4 gives an overview of the results [Cichero, 2006].

In a study of [Stroud et al., 2002], the inter- and intra-rater reliability of CA for the identification of aspirations was examined. The swallowing sounds were judged in isolation and thus the CA as an independent, stand-alone procedure was examined. The evaluation of the study resulted in a sensitivity of

Table 4. Agreement values with vs without CA used as part of the clinical swallow examination taken from [Cichero, 2006]

Agreement values	Clinical checklist without CA in %	Clinical checklist with CA in %
Sensitivity	85	89
Specificity	82	83
Positive predictive value	79	81
Negative predictive value	87	91

86%. However, specificity received a rather low percentage of 56%. The true-positive rate was indicated to be 31% and the true-negative rate to be 94% [Stroud et al., 2002]. The degree of the agreement of five therapists (inter-rater agreement) on the classification of sixteen dysphagics was only moderate (Kappa = 0.28). CA could not reliably differentiate between aspirators and non aspirators; there was a biased classification: an outsized proportion of dysphagic swallows was classified as aspirate. Individual therapists reached a high intra-rater reliability (Kappa = 0.85). The authors therefore assume that in addition to acoustic information internal, idiosyncratic criteria are used for classifying deglutition sounds. Into the same direction points the study from [Leslie et al., 2004]. Altogether the evaluations resulted in rather small intra- and inter-reliability results, which, however, are also reported with regard to the established, gold standard imaging techniques. [Leslie et al., 2004] could prove a significant connection between intra-rater reliability and sensitivity. The higher the sensitivity, the higher the intra-rater reliability. For example, i.e., the more frequently a true dysphagic is predicted correctly, the more accurate the critic is during a repeated evaluation. The authors draw the conclusion that in principle CA should permit a reliable classification. They argue, however, for the fact that classification success is, to a large part, dependent on individual skills and characteristics of the therapists and is not due to the quality of CA as a classification method. A substantial disadvantage of CA lies in the fact that there is no consensus on the underlying, physiological correlates of perceivable swallow sounds. Several sources indicate there are different theories. Some authors, e.g. [Lear et al., 1965, Logan et al., 1967,

Table 5. Variation of the number of the components of deglutition, taken from[Moriniére et al., 2006]

Number (n) of the components of deglutition	Number (n) of the recordings from 193	% %
1	3.9	2.0
2	30.9	16.0
3	87.4	45.3
4	57.9	30.0
5	11.6	6.0
6	1.0	0.5

Hamlet et al., 1992, Cichero and Murdoch, 1998], found evidence for the swallow pattern consisting primarily of two noises known as clicks or bursts. [Hamlet et al., 1992] assumes a close relationship between the change of the swallow sound and the bolus passage through the upper esophagus sphincter (UES). [Selley et al., 1994] found evidence for two clicks which are separated by a murmur. [Selley et al., 1998] and [Hamlet et al., 1992] agree on the first click is caused by the elevation of the hyolaryngeal complex. As a cause of the fine separation noise between the clicks the authors assume the passage of the bolus through UES. They attribute the second sound to the retraction of epiglottis and hyoid. [Mackowiak et al., 1967] distinguishes three parts of the swallowing sound, which he calls α, β and γ. They are interrupted by silent intervals. [Kley and Biniek, 2005] suggest still another fourth part, a δ signal, which, according to the authors, coincides with the opening of the glottis after swallowing. In healthy swallows [Cichero and Murdoch, 2003] found acoustic evidence for the glottal release sound that coincides with the subglotic air outlet in the phase after swallowing. [Moriniére et al., 2006] analyzed 193 swallow recordings of altogether 30 healthy subjects of middle age (average age: 37 ± 11 years, range: 24–63 years). Their evaluations resulted in up to six different swallow components. The number of swallow components varied both within the sample and intra-individual. The number of the most frequently shown swallow components was three (see Table 5).

[McKaig, 2002] suggests to structure the deglutition act into different landmarks, which are derived from the following phases: two bursts followed by a glottal release sound. Additionally, there is the phase of the deglutition apnea as well as a phase between the bursts, which the author calls inter-burst. All researchers agree that deglutition has an acoustic pattern. Discrepancy prevails, however, on the single components that make up this pattern. [Cichero and Langmore, 2006] suggest the metaphor of quotes and valves for a better understanding of the deglutition: deglutition can be modelled as a succession of mechanical and hydraulic actions. The authors conceive the oropharyngeal anatomy as a series of pumping and valve functions. With regard to the physiological swallow succession from proximal to distal, they propose a labial, a linguapalatal, a nasopharyngeal (soft palate), an oropharyngeal (formed out of tongue and soft palate), a laryngeal and an esophageal valve, since these structures open and close during swallowing. [Pennington and Kreutsch, 1990] make four quotes responsible for the hydraulic procedures: the oral, pharyngeal, esophageal and the respiratory pump. The oral pump stands for the retraction movement of the tongue, the pharyngeal pump for the muscle actions in the pharynx, while the bolus moves through the latter. If the esophageal valve is opened, the oesophageal pump with its peristaltic movements can begin. The last respiratory pump works not during swallowing (DA) and reinserts only after the closure release. It remains open if deglutition can be explained as a succession of the actions mentioned above. It is possible that the swallow phases are partly parallel. Taking the described model as a basis, [Cichero, 2006] suggests that the first click is caused by the closure of the laryngeal valve in conjunction with the lingual pump, which carries the bolus to the rear throat walls. Both actions induce vibrations within the pharynx, which then discharges the noise. [McKaig, 2002] assumes that first click comes about by actions which arrange the entrance of the bolus into the hypopharynx. As a trigger for the second burst [Cichero, 2006] assumes a quiet passage of the bolus through the pharynx, until a renewed vibration of the vowel tract creates a second clicking noise. The author takes mechanical opening movements as a cause for the second click of the UES in combination with pharyngeal cleaning movements. The existence of a third swallow sound has already been documented in a study by Mackowiak.[Mackowiak et al., 1967] It is yet another unsettled question whether this sound is actually another swallow sound or whether it accompanies the two clicks specified before. [Cichero and Murdoch, 2003] postulate that the final swallow sound is a result of the glottal release sound. The muscle movements during the opening of the three-level closure of the larynx set free a short air blast which accumulated in the larynx during the deglutition apnea. The authors conclude that a close relationship exists with breathings and that the final click follows the swallow, but is not an independent swallow sound. This agrees with the findings of [McKaig, 2002]. In synchronized recordings of VFES and cervical swallow sounds he was able to show that the final sound possibly escapes out of the glottis when the glottis is re-opened and coincides with the renewed onset of tidal breathing.

A recently published study by [Morinière et al., 2007] promises detailed insights. Morinière and her colleagues numerically recorded synchronized acoustic-radiologic data of 15 healthy subjects with an average age of 29.5 plus or minus 8 years [Morinière et al., 2007] to identify the origin of swallow sound components. They identify and quantify the three main swallow components with respect to the displacements of the pharyngolaryngeal structures and the bolus position from the oropharynx to the esophagus. The first sound component they found was the so called *laryngeal ascension sound* (LAS) which occures during the ascension of the hyoid bone when the bolus was located in the oropharynx and/or in the hypopharynx. The LAS was found in 81% of their recordings. In the other subjects the researchers were not able to identify a sound component that corresponded to the LAS Therefore they assume the identified sound component is frequent however albeit inconsistent in the swallow signal. Moreover it is weaker in intensity than the second main swallow component. The LAS occurs followed the study by Morinière et al. again when a number of important muscels are in a synergy contraction to move the larynx upward and forward in order to upstract the upper airway by compression. This compression is rounded out by a tip in the epiglottis. Dodds et al. assume that the displacement in the upper airway is in common with the anterosuperior movement in the hyoid [Dodds and Man, 1988]. Morinière et al. concluded, therefore, that the above mentioned movements are responsible for vibration due to contractions in the muscle fibers, rubbing in the pharyngeal and laryngeal muscle structures during heir displacements and closure of the epiglottal valve.

The second sound component Morienère et al. found is the so called *upper-sphincter opening sound* (USOS). USOS happens during the opening of the upper sphincter and at that point when the bolus passed through the sphincter. That sound the researchers found in the whole population of their subjects which indicate a constant element in the pharyngeal sound.

The last sound component located in acoustic signal is the so called laryngeal release sound (LRS) that occured when the descent and the opening of the pharynx and the larynx and when the bolus is located in the esophageus. That sound is inconsistent because it was found in only 81% of the recordings.

Of course the researcher found some movements that might be producing sounds. These are displacements of fluids, soft palate and the base of the tongue. However they cannot see what is going on behind the mandibular angle when they viewed the VFES profile. Perhaps to focus on these movements in other perspectives might give us more information on the origin of the sounds.

To sum up Morinière et al. found some evidence to define a typical profile of the pharyngeal sound with some concrete statements due to the anatomical and physiological displacements of the structures that are involved with swallowing.

Recently Leslie et al.[Leslie et al., 2007] investigated the swallow sounds in nineteen healthy subjects with a wide age range from 18 to 73. Leslie and her colleagues sought to determine: if a definitive set of swallow sounds could identify the origin of swallow sounds components like Morinière did; the order in which swallow sounds and physiologic events occur. Contradictory to the study of [Morinière et al., 2007] who obtained the cervical recording by an omidirectal microphone to conduct an acoustic-radiologic acquisition, the swallow sounds in the study of [Leslie et al., 2007] were recorded with a stethoscope and simultaneously conducting laryngoscopy and respiration monitoring. They found six sound components. However, the results were very inconsistent due to the fact that none of those sounds occured in all swallows. Moreover there were a widespread and a large degree of overlap of the timings of swallow sounds and physiologic events. The researcher found that no individual sound component could be consistently linked with a physiologic event. However [Leslie et al., 2007] have suggested four associations between swallow sound and physiologic event. First the associations between the preclick and the onset of the deglutition apnea , second the preclick is associated with the beginning of epiglottic excursion, and third the click is related to the epiglottis returning to rest. In addition the click is associated with the end of the swallow apnea.

risk of aspiration/penetration. The evaluation of CA is carried out in terms of concordance and correctness of the ratings of SLTs. The assessment of CA's validity is grounded on the sensitivity and specificity of the SLTs' ratings. In addition, in order to determine whether each classification made on the ground of CA is right or wrong, the CA outcomes are correlated with a gold standard, FEES in this case. The results did not support a statistical significance of the CA. The method stand-alone shows a poor degree intra- and inter-rater agreement (= agreement coefficient < 0.5) and low sensitivity and specificity values. Some raters yielded lower results than other SLTs. Experience with CA increases clearly the *significance* of CA judgements but the added clinical information and the video recordings increase the *predictive power* of the prognosis clearly. My study is a critical methodical evaluation of CA as an early appropriable non-invasive method in the diagnosis of dysphagia. The results demonstrate the limits of its validity.

11. Conclusion

From over 40 years of research of the method of CA there are no robust data on the sound patterns of the deglutition. But deglutition has an acoustic pattern and there are hints that the acoustic pattern, from the dyspagics is different from that of healthy ones. At present the research is not able to recommend CA as an excellent adjunct to the established dysphagia diagnosis and therapy tools in use. Today it cannot recommend establishing CA in clinical guidelines in the geriatric population. CA alone is absolutely refusable – it is not used alone in clinical practice anyway. CA as a supplement to the CSE is still doubtful and an open research question. The clinical use of CA could not be recommended. The established imaging techniques VFES and fFEES are still the only ones which are able to safely identify patients with a high penetration and aspiration risk and, above all, a silent aspiration.

Further research prospects should conduct simultaneous and blinded scoring of CA-features taking place in the videofluoroscopy.

Due to the limited view of endoscopies during the pharyngeal (White out phenomenon) and oral phase, VFES is the preferred gold standard. However, events such oral preparatory transit or movements of the upper esophagus sphincter are able to produce sounds.

Further studies should give attention to further techniques and methods that are able to support the weak CSE, for instance, measurements with EMG plus CA to develop a swallow monitoring or a combination of bronchial and cervical auscultation.

The main problem of CA is that there are high inconsistencies in the classification of the swallow sounds between the raters and even within single raters. However, some individuals reach very good results. One possibility to reduce this variability of classifications might be the creation of a checklist. With the help of precisely defined hints and instructions, the clinican assesses the clinical exam and the auscultation result. Today we are missing standardized features to give attention in the auscultation. Accordingly, it would be easier if the rater has an interpretation guideline that consists of instructions and categories. It is not entirely clear what to assess. Thus, strictly speaking, there is no CA yet! This view can be supported by the great variance of the rating results: they can be seen to bring to light that each rater has its own understanding of what CA is and hence its own CA method.

First suggestions in that direction gave us [Cichero, 2006]. A CA scheme should be evaluated for test quality in order to check if CA is more sensitive and specific in the CSE of patients with a high penetration and aspiration risk with the help of the scheme in comparison with imaging techniques.

References

[ASHA, 2000] ASHA (2000). Clinical indicators for instrumental assessment of dysphagia (guidelines). asha. *Desk Reference*, **3**:225–233.

[Böhme, 1990] Böhme, G. (1990). Ultraschalldiagnostik der zunge. *Laryngo-Rhino-Otologie*, **69**:381–388.

[Borr, 2007] Borr, C. (2007). *Zervikale Auskultation in der Dysphagie-Diagnostik– Eine Evaluationsstudie.* print and online ressource, Bielefeld University, Bielefeld.

[Borr et al., 2007] Borr, C., Hielscher-Fastabend, M., and Lücking, A. (2007). Reliability and validity of cervical auscultation. *Dysphagia*, **22**(3):225–234.

[Cichero, 2006] Cichero, J. (2006). Clinical assessment, cervical auscultation and pulse oximetry. In Cichero, J. and Murdoch, B., editors, *Dysphagia: Foundation, theory and practice*, chapter 7, page 176. John Wiley & Sons, Ltd, Chichester, New York, Weinheim, Brisbane, Toronto, Singapore.

[Cichero and Langmore, 2006] Cichero, J. and Langmore, S. (2006). Imaging assessment. In Cichero, J. and Murdoch, B., editors, *Dysphagia: Foundation, Theory and Practice*, chapter 8, pages 191–234. John Wiley & Sons, Ltd, Chichester, New York, Weinheim, Brisbane, Toronto, Singapore.

[Cichero and Murdoch, 1998] Cichero, J. and Murdoch, B. (1998). The physiologic cause of swallowing sounds: answers from heart sounds and vocal tract acoustics. *Dysphagia*, **13**:39–52.

[Cichero and Murdoch, 2002a] Cichero, J. and Murdoch, B. (2002a). Acoustic signature of the normal swallow: characterisation by age, gender and bolus volume. *Annals of Otology, Rhinology and Laryngology*, **111**(7/1):623–632.

[Cichero and Murdoch, 2002b] Cichero, J. and Murdoch, B. (2002b). Detection of swallowing sounds: methodology revisted. *Dysphagia*, **17**:40–49.

[Cichero and Murdoch, 2003] Cichero, J. and Murdoch, B. (2003). What happens after the swallow? introducing the glottal release sound. *Journal of Medical Speech Language Pathology*, **11**(1):31–41.

[Clark and Yallop, 1995] Clark, J. and Yallop, C. (1995). *An introduction to phonetics and phonology*, volume 2. Blackwell, Oxford.

[Colodny, 2000] Colodny, N. (2000). Comparison of dysphagics and nondysphagics on pulse oximetry during oral feeding. *Dysphagia*, **15**:68–73.

[Cronbach, 1951] Cronbach, L. (1951). Coefficient alpha and the internal structure of tests. *Psychometrika*, **16**:297–333.

[Daniels et al., 1997] Daniels, S., Adam, C., and Foundas, A. (1997). Clinical assessment of swallowing and prediction of dysphagia severity. *American journal of speech-language pathology*, **6**:17–24.

[DePippo et al., 1992] DePippo, K., Holas, M., and Reding, M. (1992). Validation of the 3-oz water swallow test for aspiration following stroke. *Arch Neurol*, **49**:1259–1261.

[Dodds and Man, 1988] Dodds, W. and Man, D. (1988). Influence of bolus volume on swallow-induced hyoid movementnin normal subjects. *American Journal of Radiology*, **95**:1307–1309.

[Doggett et al., 2002] Doggett, D., Turkelson, C., and Coates, V. (2002). Recent developments in diagnosis and intervention for aspiration and dysphagia in stroke and other neuromuscular disorders. *Current atherosclerosis reports*, **4**:311–318.

[Eicher et al., 1994] Eicher, P., Mano, C., and Fox, C. (1994). Impact on cervical auscultation in accuracy of clinical evaluation in predicting penetration or aspiration in a pediatric population. Minute Second Workshop on Cervical Auscultation, McLean Virginia.

[Ekberg et al., 2002] Ekberg, O., Hamdy, S., Woisard, V., Wuttge-Hannig, A., and Ortega, P. (2002). Social and psychological burden of dysphagia: its impact on diagnosis and treatment. *Dysphagia*, **17**.139–146.

[Hamlet et al., 1992] Hamlet, S., Patterson, R., Fleming, S., and Jones, L. (1992). Sounds of swallowing following total laryngectomy. *Dysphagia*, **7**:160–165.

[Hamlet et al., 1994] Hamlet, S., Penney, D., and Formolo, J. (1994). Stethoscope acoustics and cervical auscultation of swallowing. *Dysphagia*, **9**:63–68.

[Hammond et al., 2005] Hammond, L., Knutson, P., , Martino, R., Mascitelli, A., and Tebbutt, T. (2005). *Implementing a regional dysphagia management strategy: Practical considerations*. Heart and Stroke Fondation of Ontario.

[Kaplan et al., 2002] Kaplan, V., Angus, D., Griffin, M., Clermont, G., Watson, R., and Linde-Zwirble, W. (2002). Hospitalized community-acquired pneumonia in the elderly: age-and sex-related patterns of care and outcome in the united states. *Am J Respir Crit Care Med*, **165**:766–772.

[Kley and Biniek, 2005] Kley, C. and Biniek, R. (2005). Dysphagie: Sind Schluckgeräusche diagnostisch nutzbar? *Nervenarzt*, **76**:1495–1505.

[Langer, 2003] Langer, W. (2003). Methoden V: Explorative Methodenanalyse.

[Lazareck and Moussavi, 2004] Lazareck, L. and Moussavi, Z. (2004). Classification of normal and dysphagic swallows by acoustical means. *Transactions on biomedical engineering*, **51**(12):2103–2112.

[Lazareck and Moussavi, 2008] Lazareck, L. and Moussavi, Z. (access 13.01.2008). Smart algorithm for automated detection of swallowing sounds.

[Lazareck and Ramanna, 2004] Lazareck, L. and Ramanna, S. (2004). Classification of swallowing sound signals: a rough set approach. In Tsumoto, S., Slowinski, R., Komorowski, J., and Grzymala-Busse, J., editors, *Proc. of RSCTC'04, LNAI, 2066.*, pages 679–684. Springer.

[Lear et al., 1965] Lear, C., Flanagan, J., and Moorress, C. (1965). The frequency of deglutition in man. *Arch Oral Biol*, **10**:83–99.

[Leder, 2000] Leder, S. (2000). Use of arterial oxygen saturation, heart rate and blood pressure as indirect objective physiologic markers to predict aspiration. *Dysphagia*, **15**:201–205.

[Lee et al., 2006] Lee, J., Blain, S., Casas, M., Kenny, D., Berall, G., and Chau, T. (2006). A radial basis classifier for the automatic detection of aspiration in children with dysphagia. *Journal of Neuroengineering and Rehabilitation*, **3**(14).

[Leslie et al., 2004] Leslie, P., Drinnan, M., Finn, P., Ford, G., and Wilson, J. (2004). Reliability and validity of cervical auscultation: a controlled comparison using videofluoroscopy. *Dysphagia*, **19**:231–240.

[Leslie et al., 2007] Leslie, P., Drinnan, M., Zammit-Maempel, I., Coyle, J., Ford, G., and Wilson, J. (2007). Cervical auscultation synchronized with images from endoscopy swallow evaluations. *Dysphagia*, **22**(4):290–298.

[Lim et al., 2001] Lim, S., Lieu, P., Phua, S., Sesharri, R., Venketasubramanian, N., Lee, S., and Choo, P. (2001). Accuracy of bedside clinical methods compared with fiberoptic endoscopic examination of swallowing (fees) in determining the risk of aspiration in acute stroke patients. *Dysphagia*, **16**:1–6.

[Logan et al., 1967] Logan, W., Kavanagh, J., and Wornall, A. (1967). Sonic correlates of human deglutition. *J Appl Physiol*, **23**:279–284.

[Mackowiak et al., 1967] Mackowiak, R., Brenman, H., and Friedman, M. (1967). Acoustic profile of deglutition. *Proceedings of the Society for Experimental Biology*, **125**:1149–1152.

[Marik and Kaplan, 2003] Marik, P. and Kaplan, D. (2003). Aspiration pneumonia and dysphagia in the elderly. *Chest*, **124**:328–336.

[Marrie, 2000] Marrie, T. (2000). Community-acquired pneumonia in the elderly. *Clin Infect Dis*, **31**(4):1066–1078.

[Martino et al., 2000] Martino, R., Pron, G., and Diamant, N. (2000). Screening for oropharyngeal dysphagia in stroke: insufficient evidence for guidelines. *Dysphagia*, **15**:19–30.

[Mathers-Schmidt and Kurlinski, 2003] Mathers-Schmidt, B. and Kurlinski, M. (2003). Dysphagia evaluation practices: Inconsistencies in clinical assssment an instrumental examination decision-making. *Dysphagia*, **18**:114–125.

[McKaig, 2000] McKaig, T. (2000). Workshop on cervical auscultation. Florida.

[McKaig, 2002] McKaig, T. (2002). Auskultation – zervikal und thorakal. In Stanschus, S., editor, *Methoden in der klinischen Dysphagiologie*, chapter 3, pages 111–137. Schulz-Kirchner-Verlag, 1. edition.

[Moriniére et al., 2006] Moriniére, S., Beutter, P., and Boiron, M. (2006). Sound component duration of healthy human pharyngoesophageal swallowing: a gender comparison study. *Dysphagia*, **3**:175–182.

[Morinière et al., 2007] Morinière, S., Boiron, M., Alison, D., Makris, P., and Beutter, P. (2007). Origin of the sound components during pharyngeal swallowing in normal subjects. *Dysphagia*.

[Mu and Sanders, 1998] Mu, L. and Sanders, I. (1998). Neuromuscular organisation of the human upper esophageal sphincter. *Ann Otol*, **107**:370–377.

[Mueller and Lorenz, 2005] Mueller, C. and Lorenz, J. (2005). Dysphagie: Aktuelle Diagnostik und Therapie. *CME*, **2**(6):31–43.

[Oguchi et al., 2000] Oguchi, K., Saitoh, E., Baba, M., Kusudo, S., Tomomi, T., and Onogi, K. (2000). The repetitive saliva swallowing test (rsst) as a screening test of functional dysphagia (2) validity of rsst. *Jpn J Rehabil Med*, **37**:383–388.

[Pennington and Kreutsch, 1990] Pennington, G. and Kreutsch, J. (1990). Swallowing disorders: assessment and rehabilitation. *British Journal of Hospital Medicine*, **44**:17–22.

[Perlman and Schulze-Delrieu, 1997] Perlman, A. and Schulze-Delrieu, K. (1997). *Deglutition and its disorders*. Singular Publishing Group, Inc., San Diego London.

[Perry and Love, 2001] Perry, L. and Love, C. (2001). Screening for dysphagia and aspiration in acute stroke: a systematic review. *Dysphagia*, **16**:7–18.

[Reddy et al., 2000] Reddy, N., Katakam, A., Gupta, U., Unnikrishnan, R., Narayanan, J., and Canilang, E. (2000). Measurements of acceleration during videofluorographic evaluation on dysphagic patients. *Medical Engineering & Physics*, **22**(6):405–412.

[Reddy et al., 1994] Reddy, N., Thomas, R., Canilang, E., and Casterline, J. (1994). Toward classification of dysphagic patients using biomechanical measurements. *Journal of Rehabilitation Research and Development*, **31**(4):335–344.

[Richardson and Moody, 2000] Richardson, T. and Moody, J. (2000). Bedside cardiac examination: constancy in a sea of change. *Current problems in Cardiology*, **25**(11):785–825.

[Rosenbek et al., 1996] Rosenbek, J., Robbins, J., Roecker, E., Coyle, J., and Wood, J. (1996). A penetration-aspiration scale. *Dysphagia*, **11**:93–98.

[Scott et al., 1998] Scott, A., Perry, A., and Bench, J. (1998). A study of interrater reliability when using videofluoroscopy as an assessment of swallowing. *Dysphagia*, **13**:223–227.

[Sellars et al., 1998] Sellars, C., Dunnet, C., and Carter, R. (1998). A preliminary comparison of videofluoroscopy of swallow and pulse oximetry in the identificatio of aspiration in dysphagic patients. *Dysphagia*, **13**:82–86.

[Selley et al., 1998] Selley, W., Ellis, R., and Flack, F. (1998). The "cardiac hypothesis" explanation of swallowing sounds: a revision and alternative interpretation of the data. *Dysphagia*, **13**:232–234.

[Selley et al., 1994] Selley, W., Ellis, R., Flack, F., Bayliss, C., and Pearce, V. (1994). The synchronization of respiration and swallow sounds with videofluoroscopy during swallowing. *Dysphagia*, **9**:162–167.

[Sherman et al., 1999] Sherman, B., Niesenboum, J., Jesberger, B., Morrow, C., and Jesberger, J. (1999). Assessment of dysphagia with the use of pulse oximetry. *Dysphagia*, **14**:152–156.

[Smith et al., 2000] Smith, H., Lee, S., O'Neill, P., and Connolly, M. (2000). The combination of bedside swallowing assessment and oxygen saturation monitoring of swallowing in acute stroke. a safe and humane screening tool. *Age and ageing*, **29**:495–499.

[Stoeckli et al., 2003] Stoeckli, S., Huisman, T., Seifert, B., and Martin-Harris, B. (2003). Interrater reliability of videofluoroscopic swallow evaluation. *Dysphagia*, **18**:53–57.

[Stroud et al., 2002] Stroud, A., Lawrie, B., and Wiles, C. (2002). Inter- and intra-rater reliability of cervical auscultation to detect aspiration in patients with dysphagia. *Clinical Rehabilitation*, **16**:640–645.

[Takahashi et al., 1994a] Takahashi, K., Groher, M., and Michi, K. (1994a). Methodology for detecting swallowing sounds. *Dysphagia*, **9**:54–62.

[Takahashi et al., 1994b] Takahashi, K., Groher, M., and Michi, K. (1994b). Symmetry and reproducibility of swallowing sounds. *Dysphagia*, **9**:168–173.

[Vice and Bosma, 1995] Vice, F. and Bosma, J. (1995). *Cervical auscultation of feeding in adults*. University Maryland Hospitals, Baltimore, department of pediatrics edition.

[Willett, 2002] Willett, S. (2002). Cervical auscultation: objective evaluation of the swallow in normally developing 12-month-olds. Unpublished thesis for the Bachelor of Speech Pathology (honours) degree, University of Queensland.

[Youmans and Stierwalt, 2005] Youmans, S. and Stierwalt, J. (2005). An acoustic profile of normal swallowing. *Dysphagia*, **20**:195–209.

[Zenner et al., 1995] Zenner, P., Losinski, D., and Mills, R. (1995). Using cervical auscultation in the clinical dysphagia examination in long-term care. *Dysphagia*, **10**:27–31.

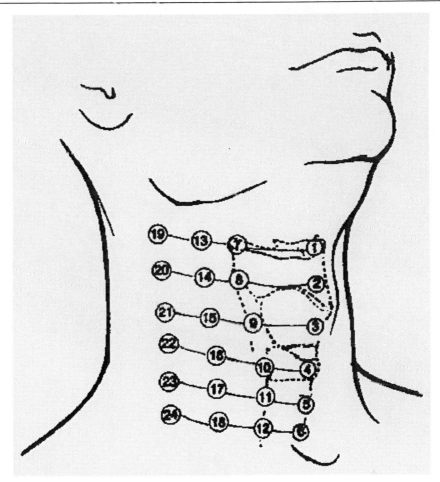

Figure 5. The 24 places of auscultation, taken from [Takahashi et al., 1994a].

In: Dysphagia   ISBN 978-1-61942-104-2
Editors: B. S. Smith and M. Adams   © 2012 Nova Science Publishers, Inc.

Chapter VII

Down's Syndrome and Dysphagia

Tracy Lazenby-Paterson
Learning Disabilities Service, NHS Lothian,
Edinburgh, UK

Abstract

Disorders of eating, drinking and swallowing (also known as 'dysphagia') commonly affect people with Down's syndrome (DS) across the lifespan. This is due to the influence of several factors, including the abnormal oral-facial features that are characteristic of the syndrome, as well as comorbid health conditions that impact on the safety and integrity of the swallowing process.

The relevant literature is consulted to explore aspects of the eating, drinking and swallowing process in people with Down's syndrome from birth onwards, and examine how this process differs from that in the general population.

Discussion focuses on how the typical eating, drinking and swallowing process in DS individuals is frequently associated with abnormal functioning of the swallowing mechanism at various levels, and how it can very often lead to dysphagia and its potentially life-threatening sequelae.

Finally, this paper considers the role of healthcare practitioners in the identification and management of dysphagia in individuals with DS, including implications for treatment planning and health service delivery.

Introduction

Dysphagia (difficulty with eating and drinking and swallowing) is a particular concern for health professionals, as it is commonly considered to be a cause of life-threatening chest illness [1]. Respiratory illness such as aspiration pneumonia is the leading cause of death amongst people with intellectual disabilities (ID), including people with Down's syndrome (DS) [2-7]. Hollins et al. [8] found that out of 2000 individuals with ID, 52% died of respiratory disease, compared with only 17% of females and 15% of males in the general population without ID.

Although the prevalence of dysphagia in people with ID is unknown, dysphagia, nutritional problems, aspiration pneumonia, respiratory illness and asphyxiation are widely considered to be more common in individuals with ID than in the general population [4-6, 9,10].

In studies of stroke patients, dysphagia was found to be an independent predictor of aspiration pneumonia, and is considered to increase risk of aspiration pneumonia by 3 to 7 times [11-14]. It is yet unclear to what extent dysphagia plays a part in the development of aspiration pneumonia in people with ID. Some studies indicate that a sole diagnosis of dysphagia is not a reliable predictor for respiratory illness. Factors such as poor oral health, a history of chest illness, the use of multiple medications, co-existing health conditions and dependency on others for feeding and oral care are also significant predictors for aspiration pneumonia [15-19].

Many of these conditions are more prevalent in people with Down's syndrome and thus increase the risk of respiratory conditions in this population. Bittles et al [20] examined the causes of death in 1332 people with Down's syndrome ranging from 0-73 years. The authors discovered a high mortality rate due to respiratory illnesses and pneumonia across all age groups, with these conditions being the most common cause of premature death in the 19-40 and 40+ age groups.

Dysphagia is commonly considered to be an important risk factor in the development of aspiration pneumonia in people with DS. Dysphagia is also a potential cause of other serious conditions, including malnutrition, obesity, dehydration and upper airway obstruction [8,11,19,21,22]

This chapter examines how the eating, drinking and swallowing process is often impaired in people with DS, and the implications of these difficulties on health service delivery.

Eating, Drinking, Swallowing and Dysphagia

In the general healthy population, the acts of eating, drinking and swallowing are typically categorised into three main events: the *oral phase*, which is subdivided into the *oral preparatory* and *oral transit* stages, the *pharyngeal phase* and the *oesophageal phase*.

Oral phase: Oral preparation begins when food enters the mouth. The lips, tongue, cheeks and jaw act together to control and hold food in the mouth, position it between the teeth, and grind it down. The grinded food mixes with saliva and once sufficiently chewed, it is collected into a cohesive mass referred to as the bolus. It is then positioned and held in a groove formed on the centre of the tongue. Oral transit begins when the anterior portion of the tongue lifts and presses against the hard palate. The mouth closes in order that the jaw can stabilise. The lips close to prevent the bolus from escaping out of the mouth, and buccal musculature ensures that food particles do not escape and collect in the spaces between the jaw and cheek. Increasingly more of the tongue pushes against the hard palate in a front-to-back direction, propelling the bolus towards the pharynx. The soft palate remains lowered and in contact with the posterior portion of the tongue to prevent premature spillage of food into the pharynx. This position of the soft palate also allows for nasal breathing during the oral phase.

The oral phase is under voluntary neural control. Therefore the amount of time taken to complete the oral phase can vary considerably according to an individual's oral motor skills, the rheological properties of food, and the preference of the individual. Upon initiation of the pharyngeal phase, all subsequent processes of the swallow are governed by involuntary reflex actions.

Pharyngeal phase: The pharyngeal swallow reflex initiates due to pressure of the bolus against the anterior faucial arches as it passes into pharynx. A build-up of air pressure is established within the oral cavity due to the closure of the lips and nasopharynx. The soft palate elevates and retracts, sealing off the nasal cavity and preventing material from entering it. Peristaltic movements push the bolus through the pharynx toward the upper oesophageal sphincter (UOS). The aryepiglottic folds, false vocal folds, and true vocal folds close to protect the airway and suspend breathing, also referred to as *swallowing apnoea*. The larynx elevates and moves forward, stretching and increasing the opening of the UOS, which also relaxes to allow the bolus to enter the oesophagus. Additional airway protection is provided by the epiglottis which lowers to cover the larynx when the bolus enters the region of the larynx. The process of coordinating breathing with swallowing is also referred to as the suck-swallow-breathe pattern.

Oesophageal phase: Once the UOS closes on the tail of the bolus, the airway reopens and breathing resumes. Peristaltic waves push the bolus down through the oesophagus towards the lower oesophageal sphincter (LOS), which opens to allow the bolus to enter the stomach [23, 24].

Dysphagia occurs due to impairment of any or all of these phases. As the organs of the swallowing system work in close coordination, if one phase is functionally impaired, the likelihood increases that other phases will also be affected [25-27].

Causes of dysphagia can include illness, injury, tumours, diseases, neurological conditions, structural problems, gastrointestinal disorders, infections and side effects of many medications [21, 28].

Eating, Drinking and Swallowing Problems in Down's Syndrome

People with DS are commonly at risk of dysphagia and its frequently life-threatening consequences. The unique structural and anatomical features typically observed in people with Down's syndrome often impinge on functioning of the eating, drinking and swallowing mechanism. In addition, many illnesses commonly observed in DS, such as congenital heart disease, dental disease, pulmonary conditions and gastroesophageal reflux disease (GORD) can also impact on the swallowing process [4, 10, 20, 29- 34]

From birth, all people with DS have systemic low tone which affects the muscles of the tongue, lips, cheeks, face, jaw, pharynx and larynx. Inadequate strength and range of muscle movement leads to reduced control and coordination of the muscles for eating, drinking and swallowing [35, 36].

Lewis et al. [37] examined the feeding problems of 20 infants with DS reported via parental questionnaire. Many of the problems observed in infants aged from 0-3 months included a weak lip seal, problems with positioning for feeding, a weak, slow and uncoordinated suck-swallow-breathe pattern and severe fatigue, all of which were associated with reduced muscle tone. Potential consequences of these difficulties included coughing, choking, aspiration, vomiting and weight loss.

The typical craniofacial characteristics of individuals with DS include a hypoplastic facial mid-third [38, 39] shortened and narrow palate [43, 44] and apparently large tongue relative to the smallness of the oral cavity [38-43].

The combination of these features and reduced muscle tone lead to tongue protrusion, mouth breathing, upper airway obstruction, malocclusion and poor coordination of breathing and swallowing [36, 37, 44, 45].

Mitchell et al. [36] performed a retrospective review of 29 children with DS ranging from 3 months to 10 years, of which 23 were diagnosed with obstructive sleep apnoea and laryngomalacia (floppy larynx). Airway obstruction and inspiratory stridor characteristic of laryngomalacia were commonly reported in these children, and are likely have a significant impact on the control of breathing and swallowing rhythm.

The large, hypotonic tongue combined with poor oral-motor skills reduces the ability of the tongue to crush food against the palate, collect food within mouth, and form a cohesive bolus. This may lead to the swallowing of inadequately chewed food, loss of food and saliva out of the mouth, and inadequate cleansing of the mouth [22].

Food and saliva loss can also occur as a consequence of malocclusion, tongue thrust, constant open mouth, poor lip control and nasal obstruction. Complications of food and saliva loss include gingivitis, tooth decay, fissuring of the tongue and lips, problems forming a cohesive bolus, and perioral infections such as *Candida albicans* [46].

There exists a very high rate of malocclusion in DS individuals due to the relationship between the underdeveloped maxilla and protruding mandible [38, 47-49]. In their review of the literature, Winter et al. [50] discovered that malocclusion was more prevalent in individuals with DS relative to the general population and other individuals with physical and intellectual disabilities such as cerebral palsy and cleft disorders.

Oral-facial dysmorphology resulting from malocclusion can significantly impair the eating, drinking and swallowing process due to poor contact between the upper and lower arches of the teeth preventing adequate grinding down and chewing of foods.

English et al. [51] examined the implications of malocclusion on chewing performance in the general population. The authors investigated chewing skills in 147 subjects with different types of malocclusion compared to 38 subjects with normal occlusion. The authors found that the subjects with malocclusion had left much larger particle sizes after chewing, and had reported more difficulty chewing harder foods than the subjects with normal occlusion. The subjects with bone class III malocclusion (underbite) experienced the greatest difficulty in both objective and subjective assessments of chewing. Although this study was performed on patients without DS, class III malocclusion is the most common malocclusion reported in people with DS [52]. DS individuals are therefore likely to experience similar difficulties to the Class III test subjects.

Studies in children and young adults with DS suggest that their underlying facial dysmorphology and malocclusion can lock the jaw and prevent adequate lateral movements for chewing [42].

Hennequin et al. [56] examined chewing ability in 11 adults with DS ranging from 17-43 years relative to 12 healthy subjects without DS. The authors discovered that DS subjects inadequately chewed their food, leading them to swallow food whole or inadequately prepared. This may lead to poor digestion, intestinal and oesophageal obstruction, and gastrointestinal problems including gastritis and ulcers [22]. A recent review also suggested that the act of swallowing food whole might lead to less satiety and leading to greater amount of food ingested [57]. This may be a potential cause for the high rates of obesity reported in DS [58-60].

Occlusal instability in DS also commonly leads to orofacial dyskinesias (abnormal and involuntary movements of the jaw and face), bruxism (persistent tooth grinding), an open mouth posture, tongue thrusting, difficulties with lip closure, and a tendency to mouth breathe. Persistent tongue protrusion also occurs as the individual with DS attempts to stabilise the jaw [54]. Difficulties with mouth and lip closure also encourage tongue protrusion in order for the DS individual to create an intraoral seal for swallowing [38, 52-55]. These features can intensify when the person with DS reaches the end of the growth period in early adulthood and can interfere with eating, drinking and swallowing [54].

In addition to malocclusion, poor muscle tone and hypermobility of the temporomandibular joints can also lead to weak and abnormal movements of the jaw and reduce chewing efficiency [61-63]. Other factors that impair chewing function include poor oral hygiene, tooth loss and periodontal disease which are more prevalent in individuals with DS [22, 55, 64-67].

Many studies suggest that DS individuals attempt to compensate for their oral-motor skill deficits by selecting soft foods that place fewer demands on chewing skills [56, 57]. Field et al. [31] examined feeding difficulties reported in the records of 349 children with and without intellectual disability ranging in age from 1 month to 12 years. They discovered a significantly higher prevalence of oral-motor problems, swallowing difficulties and texture selectivity in the 26 children with DS than in the other children without DS.

Suggested implications for texture selectivity include a reduced and restricted diet lacking in important nutrients typically found in harder and textured foods such as raw fruit and vegetables [67]. However current studies have only suggested a correlation between nutritional deficiency and poor masticatory function as opposed to a causal link [22].

Spender et al. [32] also report feeding problems in young DS children who exhibited differences in oral-motor function from typically-developing children. Such oral-motor problems include delayed initiation and poor coordination and sequencing of oral-motor movements, difficulty grading jaw movements for chewing, weak lip closure, and weak and reduced tongue movements. Other studies also find that DS children present with primitive suck patterns, poor coordination of the suck/swallow/breathe pattern, and persistent tongue protrusion [33, 68].

Problems with the pharyngeal phase of swallowing in people with DS have also been reported. Frazier et al. [33] conducted a videofluoroscopic study of oral-motor skills and swallowing function in 19 children with DS. The authors identified a disordered pharyngeal phase including delayed initiation of the pharyngeal swallow reflex in 16 of these children. 10 children aspirated on liquids, with 8 of the 10 having aspirated silently (in the absence of overt signs such as coughing).

Individuals with DS also experience problems at the oesophageal phase of swallowing. The literature reports a higher prevalence of benign oesophageal abnormalities such as atresia and tracheoesophageal fistula in children and adults with DS [69]. Other studies also reveal that oesophageal motor disorders, particularly abnormalities in oesophageal peristalsis and lower oesophageal sphincter function are more common in DS than in the general population [25, 27, 29, 30, 70-72].

In their comparative study of 58 DS adults and 38 adults without DS, Zarate et al. [30] identified a higher prevalence of achalasia in the DS subjects, symptoms of which included dysphagia for solids and liquids, regurgitation, and chest pain.

Oesophageal motor dysfunction can also lead to food loss, food refusal, gagging [31], vomiting, gastro-oesophageal reflux (GOR) [73], choking, weight loss [28], texture selectivity, and respiratory symptoms from aspiration [74-76].

In a clinical audit of 57 adults with Down's syndrome, Wallace [72] discovered that 56 of these patients presented with at least one gastrointestinal problem. Common conditions included celiac disease, achalasia, GOR, unexplained constipation or diarrhoea and over-nutrition. Over half the adults tested positive for Helicobacter Pylori infection. H. Pylori has been reported in various studies to be more prevalent in the learning disabled population, particularly those living in institutionalised settings, and can be responsible for any range of gastrointestinal symptoms such as excessive wind, GOR and vomiting [77-79].

Although the literature reports no clear association between diagnosis of DS and oesophageal carcinoma [80], Moreels et al. [81] report on 2 unusual cases of oesophageal cancer in young DS adults aged 28 and 44. Both individuals had gastro-oesophageal reflux disease, which is commonly reported in DS [31, 32, 34, 36, 82, 83], and which studies have associated with increased risk of oesophageal cancer [84].

Other co-morbid conditions commonly identified in DS children and adults include chronic pulmonary conditions, obstructive sleep apnoea and congenital heart disease. These problems can lead to food loss, food refusal, prolonged feeding times, exhaustion, gagging, vomiting, choking, difficulty progressing to more advanced textures, and increased risk of aspiration [27, 29, 30, 31, 36, 37, 73].

Maladaptive mealtime behaviours can also interfere with the eating and drinking process. Chadwick et al. [85] found that behaviours such as cramming (forcing excessive amounts of food into the mouth at once) and bolting (eating extremely quickly) were common in adults with ID, and were associated with increased risk of asphyxiation.

The literature also suggests an increased prevalence of psychiatric disorders in the DS population [112]. However Nahon et al. [115] referred to four individuals in their study whom had initially been diagnosed with eating disorders of psychogenic cause until it was discovered that they were suffering from disorders of the oesophagus. Gravestock reports several potential causes of eating disorders and abnormal eating behaviours in people with intellectual disability, including physical factors such as oral-motor problems, sensory difficulties and physical health, as well as environmental factors such as sensory deprivation and living in an institutionalised setting [113, 114].

In addition, the natural aging process brings about several changes in the structure, strength, coordination, and sensitivity of the swallowing mechanism that can directly impact on eating, drinking and swallowing function. As the life expectancy of people with DS continues to increase to beyond 60 years at present [86], DS individuals are likely to experience many of the same age-related changes as members of the general elderly population.

Gradual deterioration in muscle mass, reduced flexibility and reduced sensation of the swallowing mechanism, as well as changes in swallow-respiration coordination have been well documented as normal changes associated with aging in adults over 45 [87-93]. These changes reportedly have little functional impact on eating, drinking and swallowing in healthy elderly adults who effectively compensate for any deterioration by increasing functional output. However aging DS individuals are likely to have co-existing eating, drinking and swallowing difficulties as a consequence of their syndrome and therefore will have insufficient functional reserve to compensate for age-related changes to the swallowing mechanism. As a result, the adult with DS is likely to experience increasing difficulties with eating, drinking and swallowing as they get older, due to difficulties compensating for pre-existing swallowing problems as well as coping with any newly emerging problems.

In addition, aging DS adults are also at equal if not greater risk of developing the same illnesses and chronic conditions as the elderly general population, many of which can further impair the swallowing process [94]. These include altered dentition, xerostomia, diabetes, arthritis, stroke, malignant disease, Parkinson's disease, and dementia, all of which have been associated with coughing, choking, regurgitation, and difficulty initiating swallowing [95-97]. Many of the medications prescribed for these conditions can also lead to dysphagia [98, 99]. With several longitudinal studies confirming a premature aging process in DS adults, these conditions might also be observed at a much earlier age in people with DS [100-102].

One clinical condition, dementia of the Alzheimer's type (DAT), merits particular attention because it is well recognized that aging adults with DS are at increased risk of developing DAT than the general population [103]. Dysphagia occurs in virtually all patients with degenerative CNS diseases, including DAT, although the pattern of onset and the progression of oropharyngeal difficulties in adults suffering from DAT are currently not known [104].

In the general population, DAT causes serious impairments in motor function and coordination at both the oral and the pharyngeal phases [105], resulting in difficulties with self-feeding, chewing, initiating swallowing, managing oral secretions, nasal regurgitation, deterioration of the cough reflex, and choking [98, 104, 106]. These problems are well documented in late-stage DAT [98] and often lead to aspiration [104, 107, 108] and aspiration pneumonia [1, 19, 109] which is a major cause of death in people with DAT [110, 111].

Implications for Health Services

While there is a growing awareness that people with DS have the right to the same level of medical care and services as the general population, they are often unable to access these services largely due to a lack of understanding about dysphagia in DS and how it can be best managed [116]. Although many government reports recognise this problem [117, 118] more recent investigations confirm that adults with ID continue to experience health inequalities and discrimination in health services [119-121].

The literature proposes several causes for this. The difficulties of many DS individuals to communicate effectively and self-report symptoms can impede clinical evaluation and delay diagnosis of dysphagia [81]. DS individuals might express symptoms or pain in an atypical manner [123]. For example, Moreels et al. [81] revealed that a feeling of depression was one of the first symptoms of GOR expressed by a subject with DS.

Another cause is in relation to inadequate practitioner knowledge, skills and training about the prevalence of dysphagic conditions in DS, symptoms of dysphagia and communicative behaviours of the individual with DS. As a result, healthcare professionals may misinterpret or ignore early signs and symptoms of dysphagia [119]. If dysphagia is a symptom of an underlying disease or condition such as GORD or H Pylori, delays in evaluation, diagnosis and management can lead to more life-threatening conditions such as oesophageal cancer and potentially shorten life expectancy for people with DS [76, 78].

Several studies highlight that institutional discrimination in the healthcare setting continues to prevent adequate access to services for people with ID [120-122]. Mencap [119] investigated and reported on the premature deaths of 6 individuals with ID of whom one had a diagnosis of DS. All of the patients exhibited problems with eating, drinking or swallowing which were symptomatic of other underlying conditions. The failure to adequately address these symptoms and their underlying causes in the healthcare setting resulted in malnutrition, dehydration, aspiration pneumonia and the eventual death of these patients.

The report stresses that healthcare services fail to account for the diverse medical needs of people with ID. In addition, healthcare practitioners often rely on their own wrongful assumptions about a person's quality of life based on their own mistaken beliefs about ID, rather than taking into account presenting symptoms, patient view or the input of family and caregivers.

Diagnostic overshadowing also denies individuals with ID equity of access to healthcare. Diagnostic overshadowing refers to the failure of health professionals to accurately diagnose health problems in individuals with ID because they wrongly regard them as behavioural features inherent to the intellectual disability, and thus unsuitable for treatment [4, 126-128].

In order to address these healthcare disparities for people with DS, eating, drinking and swallowing skills should be assessed in people with DS as part of their standard health screening, alongside currently recommended screening tests such as those for thyroid conditions, congenital heart problems, and celiac disease. Roizen [129] suggests that individuals with DS would benefit from screening of a particular medical problem if they have a 10% chance of developing it, and if successful interventions exist for that problem. Various techniques are successfully used to support people with DS and eating, drinking and swallowing problems such as orthodontic procedures and specialised dental care [130], occlusal appliances [54, 131] training programmes for medical staff [131] and carers [9], texture modification [133] and environmental manipulation [9]. Regular screening for dysphagia would identify any warning signs early on and address difficulties with appropriate therapeutic techniques and treatments.

Conclusion

Current research in the literature has supported the view that from birth, people with DS suffer from many systemic and structural abnormalities and clinical conditions that impair eating, drinking and swallowing function. However there is an increasing need for further studies examining the prevalence of these problems, given that no prevalence figures of dysphagia in DS are currently available. Most current studies investigate dysphagia in a heterogeneous group of individuals with ID, or focus predominantly on eating, drinking and swallowing difficulties in small groups of children with DS.

Nonetheless it is clear from what is currently available in the literature that people with DS are at significant risk of dysphagia at some point in their lives, and that it is extremely likely that dysphagic problems will change and even worsen with age.

Dysphagia is a serious problem for many people with DS, and it can lead to life-threatening conditions such as respiratory illness, aspiration pneumonia, asphyxiation and death. Improvements in medical care, education and socioeconomic conditions have meant that the population of people with DS is increasing and living longer. However they continue to experience inequalities in access to appropriate healthcare. Difficulties with communication, poor knowledge about DS-specific disorders, and the risk of diagnostic overshadowing impede diagnosis and management of eating, drinking and swallowing problems in this population. It is essential that health care practitioners develop their understanding of the specific dysphagic problems and their signs and symptoms that can occur in this population, with the aim of predicting and identifying symptoms early on, responding proactively with timely and effective treatments, and improving health and quality of life.

References

[1]   Martin, B.; Corlew, M.; Wood, H.; Olson, D.; Golopol, L.; Wingo, M.; Kirmani, N. The association of swallowing dysfunction and aspiration pneumonia. *Dysphagia* 1994, *9(1)*, 1–6.

[2]   Cooper, S.A.; Melville, C.; Morrison, J. People with intellectual disabilities- Their health needs differ and need to be recognised and met. *BMJ* 2004, *329*, 414-415.

[3]   NHS Health Scotland. *Health needs assessment report. People with learning disabilities in Scotland;* NHS: Edinburgh, 2004.

[4]   National Patient Safety Agency. *Understanding the patient safety issues for people with learning disabilities.* NPSA: London, 2004

[5]   Stewart, L. Development of the Nutrition and Swallowing Checklist, a screening tool for nutrition and swallowing risk in people with intellectual disability. *J. Intell Dev. Disabil.* 2003, *28*, 171-187.

[6]   Carter, G.; Jancar, J. Mortality in the mentally handicapped: a 50 year survey at the Stoke Park group of hospitals (1930-1980). *J. Ment Def. Res.* 1983, *27*, 143-156.

[7]   Day, S.; Strauss, D.J.; Shavelle, R.M.; Reynolds, R.J. Mortality and causes o fdeath in persons with Down syndrome in California. *Dev. Med. Child Neurol.* 2005, *47*, 171-176.

[8]   Hollins, S.; Attard, M. T.; von Fraunhofer, N.; McGuigan, S.; Sedgwick, P. Mortality in people with learning disability: risks, causes, and death certification findings in London. *Dev. Med. Child Neurol.* 1998, *40(1)*, 50-56.

[9] Chadwick, D.; Joliffe, J.; Goldbart, J. Adherence to eating and drinking guidelines for adults with intellectual disabilities and dysphagia. *Am. J. Ment. Retard* 2003, *108(3)*, 202-211.

[10] Chadwick, D.D.; Joliffe, J. A descriptive investigation of dysphagia in adults with intellectual disabilities. *J. Intell Disabil Res.* 2009, *53(1)*, 29-43.

[11] Singh, S.; Hamdy, S. Dysphagia in stroke patients. *Postgrad. Med. J.* 2006, *82*, 383-391.

[12] Holas, M.A.; DePippo, K.L.; Reding, M.J. Aspiration and relative risk of medical complications following stroke. *Arch. Neurol.* 1994, *51*, 1051–1053.

[13] Kidd, D.; Lawson, J.; Nesbitt, R.; MacMahon J. The natural history and clinical consequences of aspiration in acute stroke. *QJM* 1995, *88*, 409–413.

[14] Mann, G.; Hankey, G.J.; Cameron, D. Swallowing function after stroke: prognosis and prognostic factors at 6 months. *Stroke* 1999, *30*, 744–8.

[15] Langmore, S.E.; Terpenning, M.S.; Schork, A.; Chen, Y.; Murray, J.T.; Lopatin, D.; Loesche, W.J. Predictors of aspiration pneumonia: how important is dysphagia? *Dysphagia* 1998, *13*, 69-81.

[16] Masiero, S.; Pierobon, R.; Previato, C.; Gomiero, E. Pneumonia in stroke patients with oropharyngeal dysphagia: a six-month follow-up study. *Neuro Sci.* 2008, *29(3)*, 139-45.

[17] Weir, K.; McMahon, S.; Barry, L.; Ware, R.; Masters, I.B.; Chang, A.B. Oropharyngeal aspiration and pneumonia in children. *Pediatr. Pulmonol.* 2007, *42*, 1024-1031.

[18] Terpenning, M. Geriatric oral health and Pneumonia Risk. *CID* 2005, 40, 1807-1810.

[19] Kikawada, M.; Iwamoto, T.; Takasaki, M. Aspiration and infection in the elderly. Epidemiology, diagnosis and management. *Drugs Aging* 2005, *22(2)*, 115-130.

[20] Bittles, A.H.; Bower, C.; Hussain, R.; Glasson, E.J. The four ages of Down syndrome. *Eur. J. Public Health* 2006, *17(2)*, 221–225.

[21] Samuels, R.; Chadwick, D.D. Predictors of asphyxiation risk in adults with intellectual disability and dysphagia. *J. Intell Disabil Res.* 2006, *50(5)*, 362-370.

[22] N'Gom, P.I.; Woda, A. Influence of impaired mastication on nutrition. *J. Prosthet Dent* 2002, *87*, 667-673.

[23] Rogers B, Arvedson J (2005) Assessment of infant oral sensorimotor and swallowing function. *Ment. Retard. Dev. Disabil Res. Rev.* 11: 74-82.

[24] Logemann, J.A. *Evaluation and Treatment of Swallowing Disorders*, 2nd edition. Pro-ed: Austin, TE, 1998, pp. 24-35.

[25] Dekel, R.; Pearson, T.; Wendel, C.; De Garmo, P.; Fennerty, M.B.; Fass, R. Assessment of oesophageal motor function in patients with dysphagia or chest pain - the Clinical Outcomes Research Initiative experience. *Aliment Pharmacol. Ther.* 2003, *18*, 1083-1089.

[26] Logemann, J.A. *Evaluation and Treatment of Swallowing Disorders*, 2nd edition. Pro-ed: Austin, TE, 1998, p 110.

[27] Triadafilopoulos, G.; Hallstone, A.; Nelson-Abbott, H.; Bedinger, K. Oropharyngeal and esophageal interrelationships in patients with nonobstructive dysphagia. *Dig. Dis. Sci.* 1992, *37(4)*, 551-557.

[28] Mittal, R.; Bhalla, V. Oesophageal motor functions and its disorders. *Gut.* 2004, *53(10)*, 1536-1542.

[29] Zárate, N.; Mearin, F. ; Gil-Vernet.; J.M. ; Camarasa, F.; Malagelada, J.R. Achalasia and Down's syndrome: coincidental association or something else? *Am. J. Gastroenterol.* 1999, *94(6)*, 1674-1677.

[30] Zárate, N.; Mearin, F.; Hidalgo, A.; Malagelada, J.R. Prospective evaluation of esophageal motor dysfunction in Down's syndrome. *Am. J. Gastroenterol.* 2001, *96 (6)*, 1718-1724.

[31] Field, D.; Garland, M.; Williams, K. Correlates of specific childhood feeding problems. *J Paediatr Child Health* 2003, *39*, 299–304.

[32] Spender, Q.; Stein, A.; Dennis, J.; Reilly, S.; Percy, E.; Cave, D. An exploration of feeding difficulties in children with Down syndrome. *Dev. Med. Child Neurol.* 1996, *38*, 681–694.

[33] Frazier, J.; Friedman, B. Swallow function in children with Down syndrome: a retrospective study. *Dev. Med. Child Neurol.* 1996, *38*, 695-703.

[34] Kerins, G.; Petrovic, K.; Bruder, M.B.; Gruman, C. Medical conditions and medication use in adults with Down syndrome: A descriptive analysis. *Downs Syndr. Res. Pract* 2007, *12(2)*, 1-7.

[35] Desai, S.S. Down syndrome: a review of the literature. *Oral Surg Oral Med Oral Pathol Oral Radiol. Endod.* 1997, *84*, 279-285.

[36] Mitchell, R.B.; Call, M.S.; Kelly, J. Ear, nose and throat disorders in children with Down Syndrome. *Laryngoscope* 2003, *113*, 259-263.

[37] Lewis, E.; Kritzinger, A. Parental experiences of feeding problems in their infants with Down syndrome. *Downs Syndr. Res. Pract* 2004, *9(2)*, 45-52.

[38] Fisher-Brandies, H. Cephalometric comparison between children with and without Down syndrome. *Eur. J. Orthodont* 1988, *10(1)*, 255-263.

[39] Dagklis, T.; Borenstein, M.; Peralta, C.F.A.; Faro, C.; Nicolaide, K.H. Three-dimensional evaluation of mid-facial hypoplasia in fetuses with trisomy 21 at 11 + 0 to 13 + 6 weeks of gestation. *Ultrasound Obstet Gynecol.* 2006, *28(3)*, 261 – 265.

[40] Austin, J.; Preger, L.; Siris, E.; Taybi, H. Short hard palate in newborn: roentgen sign of mongolism. *Radiology* 1969, *92*, 775-776.

[41] Bhagyalakshmi, G.; Renukarya, A.J.; Rajangam, S. Metric analysis of the hard palate in children with Down syndrome - a comparative study. *Downs Syndr. Res. Pract.* 2007, *12(1)*, 55-59.

[42] Hennequin, M.; Faulks, D.; Veyrune, J.L.; Bourdiol, P. Significance of oral health in persons with Down syndrome: a literature review. *Dev Med Child Neurol.* 1999, *41*, 271-283.

[43] Guimaraes, C.V.; Donnelly, L.F.; Shott, S.R.; Amin, R.S.; Kalra, M. Relative rather than absolute macroglossia in patients with Down syndrome: implications for treatment of obstructive sleep apnea. *Pediatr. Radiol.* 2008, *38(10)*, 1062-1067.

[44] Nargozian, C. The airway in patients with craniofacial abnormalities. *Pediatr Anesth* 2004, *14*, 53-59.

[45] Boston, M.; Rutter, M. Current airway management in craniofacial anomalies. *Curr. Opi. Otolaryngol. Head Neck Surg.* 2003, *11*, 428-432.

[46] Meningaud, J.P.; Poramate, R.A.; Chikhani, L.; Bertrand, J.C. Drooling of saliva: A review of the etiology and management options. *Oral Surg Oral Med. Oral Pathol Oral Radiol Endod.* 2006, *101(1), 48-57.

[47] Cohen, M.M.; Winer, R.A. Dental and facial characteristics in Down's syndrome (Mongolism). *J. Dent Res.* 1965, *44*, 197-208.

[48] Kisling, K. Craneal morphology in Down's syndrome. A comparative roentencephalometric study in adults males. *Munksgaard* 1960, *107*, 90-98.

[49] Oliveira, A.C.; Paiva, S.M.; Campos, M.R.; Czeresnia, D. () Factors associated with malocclusions in children and adolescents with Down syndrome. (Online only) *Am. J. Orthod Dentofacial Orthop* 2008, *489*, e1-e8.

[50] Winter, K.; Baccaglini, L.; Tomar, S. A review of malocclusion among individuals with mental and physical disabilities. *Spec. Care Dentist* 2008, *28(1)*, 19-26.

[51] English, J.D.: Buschang, P.H.; Throckmorton, G.S. Does malocclusion affect masticatory performance? *Angle Orthod* 2002, *72(1)*, 21-27.

[52] Alió-Sanz, J.J. A new cephalometric diagnostic method for Down's Syndrome patients with open bite. *Med. Oral Patol Oral Cir. Bucal.* 2008, *1,13(3)*, E171-5

[53] Haw, C.; Barnes, T.; Clark, K.; Crichton, P.; Kohen, D. Movement disorder in Down's syndrome: a possible marker of the severity of mental handicap. *Mov. Dis* 1996, *11(4)*, 395–403.

[54] Faulks, D.; Veyrune, J.L.; Hennequin, M. Consequences of oral rehabilitation on dyskinesia in adults with Down's syndrome: a clinical report. *J. Oral Rehabil.* 2002, *29*, 209-218.

[55] Hennequin, M; Allison, P.J.; Veyrune, J.L. Prevalence of oral health problems in a group of individuals with Down syndrome in France. *Dev Med. Child Neurol.* 2000, *42*, 691-698.

[56] Hennequin, M.; Allison, P.J.; Faulks, D.; Orliaguet, T.; Feine, J. Chewing indicators between adults with Down syndrome and controls. *J. Dent Res.* 2005, *84(11)*, 1057-1061.

[57] Faulks, D.; Collado, V.; Mazille, M.N.; Veyrune, J.L.; Hennequin, M. Masticatory dysfunction in persons with Down's syndrome. Part 1: aetiology and incidence. *J. Oral Rehabil* 2008, *35(11)*, 854-862.

[58] Delrue, M.A.; Michaud, J.L. Fat chance: genetic syndromes with obesity. *Clin. Genet* 2004, *66*, 83-93.

[59] Prasher, V.P. Overweight and obesity amongst Down's syndrome adults. *J. Intell Disabil Res.* 1995, *39*, 437-441.

[60] Braunschweig, C.L.; Gomez, S.; Sheean, P.; Tomey, K.M.; Rimmer, J.; Heller, T. Nutritional status and risk factors for chronic disease in urban-dwelling adults with Down syndrome. *Am. J. Ment. Retard.* 2004, *109*, 186-193.

[61] Sato, S.; Ohta, M.; Goto, S.; Kawamura, H.; Motegi, K. Electromyography during chewing movement in patients with anterior disc displacement of the temporomandibular joint. *Int. J. Oral Maxillofac Surg* 1998, *27*, 274-277.

[62] Bhowate, R.; Dubey, A. Dentofacial changes and oral health status in mentally challenged children. *J. Indian Soc. Pedod. Prev. Dent* 2005, *23(2)*, 71-73.

[63] Woda A.; Mishellany, A.; Peyron, M.A. The regulation of masticatory function and food bolus formation. *J. Oral Rehabil.* 2006, *33*, 840-849.

[64] Helm, S.; Petersen, P.E. Causal relation between malocclusion and periodontal health. *Acta Odontol. Scand.* 1989, *47*, 223-228.

[65] Oredugba, F. Oral health condition and treatment needs of a group of Nigerian individuals with Down syndrome. *Downs Syndr. Res. Pract.* 2007, *12(1)*, 72-77.

[66] Gabre, P.; Martinsson, T.; Gahnberg, L. Longitudinal study of dental caries, tooth mortality and interproximal bone loss in adults with intellectual disability. *Eur J Oral Sci* 2001, *109*, 20-26.

[67] Waldman, H.B.; Perlman, S.P.; Swerdloff, M. Orthodontics and the population with special needs. *Am. J. Orthod Dentofacial. Orthop* 2000, *118*, 14-17.

[68] Glatz-Noll, E.; Berg, R. Oral dysfunction in children with Down syndrome: an evaluation of treatment effects by means of videoregistration. *Eur. J. Orthod* 1991, *31*, 446–451.

[69] Bianca, S.; Bianca, M,; Ettore, G. Oesophageal atresia and Down syndrome. *Downs Syndr. Res. Pract.* 2002, *8(1)*, 29-30.

[70] Boeckxstaens, G.; Jonge, W.; van den Wijngaard, R.; Benninga, M. Achalasia: From new insights in pathophysiology to treatment. *J. Pediatr. Gastroenterol. Nutr.* 2005, *41(1)*, S36-S37.

[71] Okawada, M.; Okazaki, T.; Yamataka, A.; Lane, G.J.; Miyano, T. Down's syndrome and esophageal achalasia: a rare but important clinical entity. *Pediatr Surg. Int.* 2005, *21*, 997-1000.

[72] Wallace, R.A. Clinical audit of gastrointestinal conditions occurring among adults with Down syndrome attending a specialist clinic. *J. Intell Dev. Disabil.* 2007, *32*, 45-50.

[73] Marder, E.; Dennis, J. Medical management of children with Down's syndrome. *Curr. Paediatr.* 2001, *11*, 57–63.

[74] Roizen, N.; Patterson, D. Down's syndrome. *Lancet* 2003, *361*,1281–1289.

[75] Seddon, P.C.; Khan, Y. Respiratory problems in children with neurological impairment. *Arch. Dis. Child* 2003, *88(1)*, 75–78.

[76] Prakash, C.; Clouse, R.E. Esophageal motor disorders. *Curr. Opin. Gastroenterol.* 2002, *18*, 454-463.

[77] Beange, H.; Lennox, N. Physical aspects of health in the learning disabled. *Curr. Opin. Psychiatry* 1998, *11*, 531–534.

[78] Duff, M.; Scheepers, M.; Cooper, M.; Hoghton, M.; Baddeley, P. Helicobacter pylori: Has the killer escaped from the institution? A

possible cause of increased stomach cancer in a population with intellectual disability. *J. Intell Disabil Res.* 2001, *45(3)*, 219-225.

[79] Morad, M.; Merrick, J.; Nasri, Y. Prevalence of Helicobacter pylori in people with intellectual disability in a residential care centre in Israel. *J. Intell Disabil. Res.* 2002, *46(2)*, 141-143.

[80] Hill, D.A.; Gridley, G.; Cnattingius, S.; Mellemkjaer, L.; Linet, M.; Adami, H.O.; Olsen, J.H.; Nyren, O.; Fraumeni, J.F. Jr. Mortality and cancer incidence among individuals with Down syndrome. *Arch. Intern. Med.* 2003, *163*, 705-711.

[81] Moreels, T.G.; van Vliet, E.P.M.; Tilanus, H.W.; Tran, T.C.K.; Kuipers, E.J.; Siersema, P.D. Down syndrome and esophageal cancer. *Dis. Esophagus* 2007, *20*, 183-186.

[82] Bohmer, C.J.; Klinkenberg-Knol, E.C.; Niezen-de Boer, M.C.; Meuwissen, S.G. Gastroesophageal reflux disease in intellectually disabled individuals: how often, how serious, how manageable? *Am. J. Gastroenterol.* 2000, *95*, 1868-1872.

[83] Carr, M.; Nguyen, A.; Nagy, M.; Poje, C.; Pizzuto, M.; Brodsky, L. Clinical presentation as a guide to the identification of GERD in children. *Int. J. Pediatr. Otorhinolaryngol* 2000, *54*, 27-32.

[84] Lagergren, J. Adenocarcinoma of oesophagus: what exactly is the size of the problem and who is at risk? *Gut* 2005, *54*, (Suppl I) il-5.

[85] Chadwick, D.D.; Samuels, R. Predictors of asphyxiation risk in adults with intellectual disabilities and dysphagia. *J. Intell Disabil. Res.* 2006, *50(5)*, 362-370.

[86] Glasson, E.J.; Sullivan, S.G.; Hussain, R.; Petterson, B.A.; Montgomery, P.D.; Bittles A.H. The changing survival profile of people with Down's syndrome: implications for genetic counselling. *Clin. Genet* 2002, *62*, 390–393.

[87] Jaradeh, S. Neurophysiology of swallowing in the aged. *Dysphagia* 1994, *9(4)*, 218–220.

[88] Fucile, S.; Wright, P.M.; Chan, I.; Yee, S.; Langlais, M.E.; Gisel, EG. Functional oral-motor skills: do they change with age? *Dysphagia* 1998, *13*, 195–201.

[89] Volpi, E.; Nazemi, R.; Fujita, S.; Muscle tissue changes with aging. *Curr Opin Clin. Nutr. Metab. Care* 2004, *7*, 405–410.

[90] Nicosia, M.; Hind, J.; Roecker, E.; Carnesm M.; Doylem J.; Dengelm G.; Robbinsm J. Age effects on the temporal evolution of isometric and swallowing pressure. *J. Gerontol.* 2000, *55A(11)*, M634–M640.

[91] Peyron, M.A.; Blanc, O.; Lund, J.P.; Woda, A. Influence of age on adaptability of human mastication. *J. Neurophysiol.* 2004, 92, 773–779.

[92] Barczi, S.; Sullivan, P.; Robbins, J. How should dysphagia care of older adults differ? Establishing optimal practice patterns. *Semin. Speech Lang* 2000, *21(4)*, 347–363.

[93] Robbins, J.; Gangnon, R.; Theis, S.; Kays, S.; Hewitt, A.; Hind, J. The effects of lingual exercise on swallowing in older adults. *J. Am. Geriatr. Soc.* 2005, *53*, 1483–1489.

[94] Kawashima, K.; Motohashi, Y.; Fujishima, I. Prevalence of dysphagia among community-dwelling elderly individuals as estimated using a questionnaire for dysphagia screening. *Dysphagia* 2004, *19*, 266–271.

[95] Martin-Harris, B.; Brodsky, M.B.; Michel, Y.; Ford, C.; Walters, B.; Heffner, J. Breathing and swallowing dynamics across the adult lifespan. *Arch. Otolaryngol. Head Neck Surg* 2005, *131(9)*, 762–770.

[96] Hirst,L.; Ford, G.; Gibson, G.; Wilson, J. Swallow-induced alterations in breathing in normal older people. *Dysphagia* 2002,17, 152–161.

[97] Achem, S.; DeVault, K. Dysphagia in aging. *J. Clin. Gastroenterol.* 2005, *39(5)*, 357–371.

[98] Priefer, B.; Robbins, J. Eating changes in mild-stage Alzheimer's disease: a pilot study. *Dysphagia* 1997, 12(4), 212–221.

[99] Morris, H. Dysphagia in the elderly - a management challenge for nurses. *Br. J. Nurs.* 2006, *15(10)*, 558–562.

[100] Holland, A.J. Down's Syndrome. In *Dementia, Aging, and Intellectual Disabilities: A Handbook;* Janicki, M.; Dalton, A.; Eds; Brunner/Mazel: New York, NY, 1998, pp 184–185.

[101] Carmeli, E.; Kessel, S.; Bar-Chad, S.; Merrick, J. A comparison between older persons with Down syndrome and a control group: Clinical characteristics, functional status and sensorimotor function. *Downs Syndr Res Pract* 2004, *9(1)*, 17–24.

[102] Burt, D.; Primeaux-Hart, K.; Loveland, K.; Cleveland, L.; Lewis, K.; Lesser, J.; Pearson, P. Aging in adults with intellectual disabilities. *Am. J. Ment. Retard* 2005, *110(4)*, 268–284.

[103] Bush, A.; Beail, N. Risk factors for dementia in people with Down syndrome: issues in assessment and diagnosis. *Am. J. Ment Retard.* 2004, *109(2)*, 83–97.

[104] Wada, H.; Nakajoh, K.; Satoh-Nakagawa, T.; Suzuki, T.; Ohrui, T.; Arai, H.; Sasaki, H. Risk factors of aspiration pneumonia in Alzheimer's disease patients. *Gerontology* 2001, *47*, 271–276.

[105] Silverman, W.; Zigman, W.; Huykang, K.; Krinsky-McHale, S.; Wisniewski, H. Aging and dementia among adults with mental retardation and Down Syndrome. *Top. Geriatr Rehabil* 1998, *13(3)*, 49–64.

[106] Buchholz, D.; Robbins, J. Neurologic diseases affecting oropharyngeal swallowing. In *Deglutition and Its Disorders- Anatomy, Physiology, Clinical Diagnosis and Management;* Perlman, A.; Schulze-Delrieu, K.; Eds.; Singular: San Diego, CA, 1997; pp 326–327.

[107] Horner, J.; Alberts, M.; Dawson, D.; Cook, G. Swallowing in Alzheimer's disease. *Alzheimer Dis. Assoc Disord.* 1994, *8(3)*, 177–189.

[108] Kalia, M. Dysphagia and aspiration pneumonia in patients with Alzheimer's disease. *Metabolism* 2003, *52(10)*, 36–38.

[109] Loeb, M.; McGeer, A.; McArthur, M.; Walter, S.; Simor, A. Risk factors for pneumonia and other lower respiratory tract infections in elderly residents of long-term care facilities. *Arch. Intern. Med.* 1999, *159(17)*, 2058–2064.

[110] Marik, P.; Kaplan, D. Aspiration pneumonia and dysphagia in the elderly. *Chest* 2003, *124(1)*, 328–336.

[111] Ganguli, M.; Dodge, H.; Shen, C.; Pandav, R.; DeKosky, S. Alzheimer disease and mortality: a 15-year epidemiological study. *Arch. Neurol.* 2005, *62(5)*, 779–784.

[112] Myers, B.; Pueschel, S. Psychiatric disorders in persons with Down syndrome. *Journal Nerv. Men. Dis.* 1991, *179(10)*, 609-613.

[113] Gravestock, S. Eating disorders in adults with intellectual disability. *J. Intell Disabil. Res.* 2000, *44(6)*, 625-637.

[114] Gravestock, S. Diagnosis and classification of eating disorders in adults with intellectual disability: the Diagnostic Criteria for Psychiatric Disorders for Use with Adults with Learning Disabilities/Mental Retardation (DC-LD) approach. *J. Intell Disabil. Res.* 2003, *47(1)*, 72-83.

[115] Nahon, S.; Boudet, MJ.; Godeberge, P.; Mal, F.; Lévy, P.; Perniceni. T.; Gayet, B. Achalasie mimant des troubles du comportement alimentaire. *Gastroenterol. Clin. Biol.* 2001, *25*, 313-315.

[116] Disability Rights Commission (DRC). *Equal treatment: Closing the gap. A formal investigation into the physical health inequalities experienced by people with learning disabilities and/or mental health problems;* Disability Rights Commission: London, 2006.

[117] Department of Health. *Valuing people: A new strategy for learning disabilities for the 21st Century*; Department of Health: London, 2001

[118] Scottish Executive. *The same as you? A review of services for people with learning disabilities*; Scottish Government: Edinburgh, 2000.

[119] Mencap. *Death by Indifference, Following up the Treat me right! Report*. Mencap: London, 2007.

[120] Michael, Sir J, *Healthcare for all: Report of the independent inquiry into access to healthcare for people with learning disabilities*. London, July 2008.

[121] House of Lords, House of Commons Joint Committee on Human Rights. *A Life Like Any Other? Human Rights of Adults with Learning Disabilities*, Seventh Report of Session 2007–08, Vol 1.

[122] Healthcare Commission. *A life like no other: a national audit of specialist inpatient healthcare services for people with learning difficulties in England*; December 2007.

[123] Hennequin, M. ; Morin, C. ; Feine, J.S. Pain expression and stimulus localization in individuals with Down's syndrome. *Lancet* 2000, *356*, 1882-1887.

[124] Puri, B.K.; Lekh, S.K.; Langa, A.; Zaman, R.; Singh, I. Mortality in a hospitalized mentally handicapped population: a 10-year survey. *J. Intell Disabil Res.*, 1995, *39*, 442-446.

[125] Kmietowicz, Z. Down's children received "less favourable" hospital treatment. *BMJ* 2001, *322*, 815.

[126] Reiss, S.; Levitan, G.W.; Szysko, J. Emotional disturbance and mental retardation: diagnostic overshadowing. *Am. J. Ment. Def.* 1982, *86*, 567-574.

[127] Mason, J.; Scior, K. 'Diagnostic overshadowing' amongst clinicians working with people with intellectual disabilities in the UK. *J. App. Res. Intell Disabil.* 2004, *17*, 85-90.

[128] Leslie, P.; Crawford, H.; Wilkinson, H. People with a Learning Disability and Dysphagia: A Cinderella Population? *Dysphagia* 2008, in press.

[129] Roizen, N. The early interventionist and the medical problems of the child with Down syndrome. *Inf. Young Child* 2003, *16(1)*, 88-95.

[130] Musich, D.R. Orthodontic intervention and patients with Down syndrome. The role of inclusion, technology and leadership. *Angle Orthod* 2006, *76(4)*, 734-735.

[131] Mazille, M.N.; Woda, A.; Nicolas, E.; Peyron, M.A.; Hennequin, M. Effect of occlusal appliance wear on chewing in persons with Down syndrome. *Physiology Behavior.* 2008, *93*, 919-929.

[132] Rosenvinge, S.; Starke, I. Improving care for patients with dysphagia. *Age Ageing* 2005, *34(6)*, 587-593.

[133] Logemann, J.A. *Evaluation and Treatment of Swallowing Disorders*, 2nd edition. Pro-ed: Austin, TE, 1998, pp 202-203.

Index

N

O

P